Series in Laboratory Medicine
Leo P. Cawley, M.D., Series Editor

Clinical Laboratory Statistics, Second Edition
Roy N. Barnett, M.D.

Electrophoresis and Immunoelectrophoresis
Leo P. Cawley, M.D.

Laboratory Diagnostic Procedures in the Rheumatic Diseases, Second Edition
Alan S. Cohen, M.D.

Practical Blood Transfusion, Second Edition
Douglas W. Huestis, M.D., Joseph R. Bove, M.D.,
Shirley Busch, M.P.H., SBB (ASCP)

Exfoliative Cytopathology, Second Edition
Zuher M. Naib, M.D.

Immunopathology: Clinical Laboratory Concepts and Methods
Robert M. Nakamura, M.D.

Laboratory Management
Jack E. Newell, M.D.

The Diagnosis of Bleeding Disorders, Second Edition
Charles A. Owen, Jr., M.D., Ph.D., E. J. Walter Bowie, M.A., B.M., F.A.C.P.,
John H. Thompson, Jr., Ph.D.

Serum Protein Abnormalities: Diagnostic and Clinical Aspects
Stephan E. Ritzmann, M.D., Jerry C. Daniels, M.D., Ph.D.

Histopathology of the Bone Marrow
Arkadi M. Rywlin, M.D.

Laboratory Procedures in Clinical Microbiology
John A. Washington II, M.D.

Clinical Laboratory Statistics

Clinical Laboratory Statistics

Second Edition

Roy N. Barnett, M.D.
Clinical Professor of Pathology,
Yale University School of Medicine, New Haven;
Chairman, Pathology Service, Norwalk Hospital,
Norwalk, Connecticut

With contributions by IRWIN M. WEISBROT, M.D.
Associate Clinical Professor of Pathology,
Yale University School of Medicine, New Haven;
Senior Attending Pathologist, Norwalk Hospital,
Norwalk, Connecticut

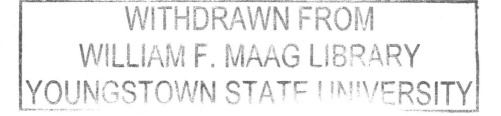
Little, Brown and Company
Boston

To Margaret Barnett
my deep appreciation for assistance
in the slow process of creating this volume

Preface

This volume is intended for the many persons who are intimately concerned with clinical laboratory problems and who require an understanding of statistics to help them cope with those problems. Although the statistical treatment is too elementary to instruct an accomplished statistician, and the clinical and laboratory information is too superficial for the education of pathologists, I hope that the bringing together of both the medical laboratory and the statistical viewpoints will be enlightening.

The material is arranged in five parts: (1) Principles of Statistical Analysis defines and explains those terms most often employed in medical laboratory statistics and outlines the usual form of their application. (2) Application of Statistics in the Clinical Laboratory describes specific applications in developing and maintaining a good laboratory. (3) Application of Statistics in Patient Care incorporates material relevant to laboratory tests for sick patients, apparently well persons, and population groups. (4) Statistics for Manufacturers describes techniques useful for validating the performance of various laboratory products. (5) Statistics in Medical Literature is a brief discussion of good and poor practices often characterizing statistical presentations in scientific discourse.

Considerable new material has been added since the first edition, for theoretical background information and because of our additional practical experience. It includes chi-square for multiple variables; Poisson distribution; use of median values; a chapter on linear regression; normal values; quality control in hematology; interference studies; precautions to follow in method comparison studies; a chapter on computers in the laboratory, indicating their role in applying statistical concepts; and a chapter on statistics for manufacturers, particularly directed toward meeting requirements of the Food and Drug Administration. Several tables made unnecessary by today's simple electronic calculators have been dropped, and a new table for computing one-sided confidence limits for σ has been added.

The appendix tables bring together commonly used reference values. Finally, there are a few general references listed for those who wish to pursue statistical studies further.

For doing the required arithmetic a pocket calculator or larger device capable of extracting square roots and performing other standard manipulations is necessary; many inexpensive models are available. Ordinary graph paper and a good straightedge are worthwhile to depict figures graphically. For repetitive tasks or complex calculations a programmable calculator is invaluable, particularly if it provides printed results for a permanent record.

I make no claim that this is a comprehensive or authoritative treatise. (Professor A. A. Liebow says, "An authority is someone who can't learn any more," and I have lots to learn.) I do hope that this somewhat enlarged second edition will continue to be helpful to practical laboratorians.

I acknowledge my debt to all who helped me to learn about statistical applications. My particular mentor was the late Dr. W. J. Youden, who contributed the Foreword to the first edition. He was incredibly patient in answering questions. How often I wish he were still available to solve the problems which I find impossible but which he would have conquered in a moment! I am grateful to Irwin M. Weisbrot, M.D., my longtime associate, whose new contributions in this edition are a necessary and welcome addition. The advice of Domenic V. Cicchetti, Ph.D., on numerous aspects of statistics, and the help of V. J. Kambli, Ph.D., with calculations and chemical data, were most valuable.

My thanks to Mrs. Virginia Simon, medical illustrator at the Yale University School of Medicine, for the high caliber of the illustrations she prepared, and to John L. Meyer II, M.D., pathologist of the Day Kimball Hospital, Putnam, Connecticut, for the delightful cartoons.

My apologies to my family and friends for ignoring them while I labored over this work. My particular gratitude goes to my wife, who did all the typing and manuscript preparation.

R.N.B.

Foreword to the First Edition

The constant increase in laboratory tests, both in numbers and in variety, has made the clinical laboratory an ever more significant part of the medical scene. It has also made statistical analysis a vital factor in evaluating the results of these tests, whether they are run by means of highly automated equipment or simple "kits." The level of a test value that might serve to initiate medical or surgical action may be obscured by the use of an inaccurate or a biased test method.

An outstanding feature of Dr. Barnett's book is the emphasis placed on the adequacy of test methods. It is not enough to get concordant results in one laboratory using one test method. Such results, if biased, may have a purely local and temporary usefulness, no longer acceptable in our mobile era. Satisfactory methods should give values as close to the chemist's "correct" value as possible. They should yield reproducible results by different operators in different laboratories at different times. Furthermore, the measurement error should be small when compared with the range of values encountered among healthy individuals. Various means of checking the accuracy and bias of specific methods are discussed here in detail.

Dr. Barnett also explains the use and advantage of quality control charts for these methods. These charts provide a visual guide of day-to-day variation for the attending physician, enabling him to achieve quickly an awareness of which fluctuations in patients results are without medical significance and which are meaningful.

This practical volume gives an account of years of laboratory work directed to the evaluation and comparison of test procedures. It is thus a very personal book, as useful for the great mass of statistical detail that is omitted as for the extremely useful material included.

W. J. Youden

Contents

III. Application of Statistics in Patient Care

IV. Statistics for Manufacturers

V. Statistics in Medical Literature

Appendix Tables

I Principles of Statistical Analysis

Statistical Abbreviations for Laboratory Use

ANOVA	analysis of variance
χ^2	chi-square
CI	confidence interval
CV	coefficient of variation
Δ	delta
$\bar{d}$	average difference
df	degrees of freedom
F	F test for variance
μ	mean of the population
n	number of values
p	probability level
P	percentile
r	correlation coefficient
s	standard deviation of a sample
s^2	variance, the square of the standard deviation
SE	standard error
$S_{y \cdot x}$	standard deviation of y on x
σ	standard deviation of the population
Σ	sum of
t	t test for comparing means
$\bar{x}$	mean of a sample

1 Terminology

Statistics may be defined as the science of dealing with groups of numbers.* As a general procedure a series of numbers is acquired, the numbers are related to each other in some way, and then information is derived from their relationships. This information furnishes some sort of generality whose validity can then be determined.

In order to understand the statistician's approach, it is necessary to define some of the concepts that are frequently used.

Population
The population is the group of individual values about which we hope to derive a generalization. It must be clearly defined. Examples: all 14-year-old American males; all fiberglass outboard cruisers.

Sample
The sample is the group of individual values actually studied. It is essential that it be representative if it is to be used for estimating the values for the whole population. If everything else is equal, the larger the sample the more likely it is to provide a good estimate of the population. For example, if we wish to generalize about the height of 14-year-old boys in Henry Hudson School in Rye, New York, and we actually measure the height of all members of this group, our knowledge of the population distribution for various heights is extremely accurate. However, if we measure the same group and attempt to estimate from it the heights of all the 14-year-old boys in New York State or the United States or the world, the sample would become increasingly inadequate as the population enlarged. Such factors as race distribution and early dietary habits would assume a larger role as our population increased.

Curve of Normal Distribution
The curve of normal distribution (Figure 1-1) is a symmetrical bell-shaped curve representative of many types of numerical distributions. (The term *normal* is not used here in the common medical sense, e.g., a normal person is one free from disease or abnormality.) This curve has a standard shape which can be found by using an expansion of the binomial theorem $(p + q)^n$; it has many

*The *Random House Dictionary of the English Language* definition reads: **sta·tis·tics** . . . *n* 1. (*construed as sing.*) the science that deals with the collection, classification, analysis, and interpretation of numerical facts or data, and that, by use of mathematical theories of probability, imposes order and regularity on aggregates of more or less disparate elements. 2. (*construed as pl.*) the numerical facts or data themselves. (From the *Random House Dictionary of the English Language*, The Unabridged Edition, Copyright © 1966, 1973 by Random House, Inc. Reprinted by permission.)

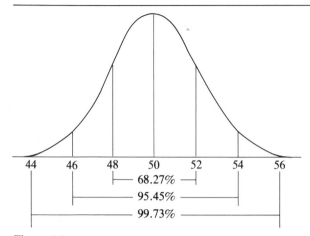

Figure 1-1
Curve of normal distribution. Mean = 50; s = 2. Percentages are the percentage of the area under the curve described by multiples of the standard deviation.

uses in statistics. It is also called the Gaussian curve or the curve of De Moivre, Bernoulli, Laplace, and Gauss.

Standard Deviation

The standard deviation is a measure of the dispersion of a group of values around a mean. Indicated by s (some authors use SD), it is derived from the curve of normal distribution and bears a meaningful relation to the area under the normal distribution curve so that, for example, the area under the center of the curve represented by the mean $\pm$ 2s is 95.45 percent of the whole area. Standard deviation is expressed in absolute units, such as milligrams per 100 ml. The symbol σ denotes the standard deviation of the whole population, whereas s denotes the standard deviation of the sample studied.

$S_{y \cdot x}$ is the standard deviation of data points scattered about a line. The line may be regarded as a mean ($\bar{x}$) and $S_{y \cdot x}$ as the standard deviation of the data points.

Coefficient of Variation

The coefficient of variation (CV) is another way of expressing standard deviation. It is defined as 100 times the standard deviation divided by the mean; it is expressed as a percentage. Its chief value is that it relates the standard deviation to the level at which the measurements are made. For example, a variability of 1 mm. (1 standard deviation) in measuring a 5 mm. object (CV = 20%) is very different from the same variability of 1 mm. in measuring a 5 meter distance (CV = .02%).

Confidence Limits

Confidence limits are limits between which we expect a specified proportion of a population to lie with respect to a measured characteristic. For instance, we might say that 95 percent of a group of normal individuals have fasting blood glucose levels of 85 to 128 mg. per 100 ml.; our 95 percent confidence limits are then 85 and 128.

Confidence Interval

The confidence interval (CI) is the interval within which we may be reasonably confident that the true population lies when values are determined from a small sample of that population.

Mean Deviation

The mean deviation is a rarely used figure. It is found by taking the difference of each measurement from the average for the whole set, without regard to sign, and dividing by the number of measurements. The standard deviation is much more useful.

Standard Error

The standard error (SE) is a measure of the dispersion of the *mean* of a set of measurements. It is therefore smaller than the standard deviation of a single series of measurements from the same population. It is used to *compare means* with one another and is calculated by dividing the standard deviation by the square root of the number of determinations.

Range

Range is another measure of dispersion of values and is merely the difference between the largest and smallest of a group of measurements. It is generally less useful for its intended purpose than is the standard deviation.

Variance

Variance (s^2) is the square of the standard deviation. (In actually calculating s we first find s^2 and then take its square root.) It has the mathematical advantage over s that variances can be added or subtracted, which standard deviations cannot, so that when we attempt to assign numerical values to different components affecting inherent variability, we perform an *analysis of variance* (ANOVA).

Percentile

Percentile (P) is another measure of dispersion of a series of numbers. It is expressed as the percentage of numbers falling below a certain figure and is often written as $P_{subscript}$. Example: $P_{90} = 12$ indicates that 90 percent of observed values are 12 or less.

Probability

Probability level (p) is used by statisticians in evaluating the results of their manipulations. It refers to the probability that a figure equal to or larger than the one obtained would occur by chance alone. It is now usually expressed in decimal form, so .20 means the odds are 20 *in* 100, or 1 *to* 4, or 20 percent. For example, if a statistical test result is significant at the .05 probability level (p = .05), this signifies that such a value would occur by chance alone less than 5 times in 100 trials.

Significance Level

It is frequently desirable to choose an arbitrary cutoff level for probability. We may decide that in the context of our analysis a probability of .20 is not significant but .05 is significant. The usual cutoff levels are .05, often termed *significant,* and .01, often termed *highly significant.* Convenient tables are available for various-sized samples at each of these levels.

Mean

The mean or arithmetic mean or average ($\bar{x}$, pronounced "x bar") is the numerical mean value calculated for a series of numbers. μ is the mean of the entire population from which the sample is drawn.

Median

The median is another measurement of the center of a distribution. It is defined as the point on the scale that has equal numbers of observations above and below it.

Mode

The mode is still another measurement of the center of a distribution. It is defined as the value that occurs most frequently.

Σ

Σ (Greek capital letter sigma) is the symbol used to express "the sum of." It is frequently complicated by the addition of subscripts and superscripts. The superscript gives the number of observations; the subscript, the intervals. Example:

$$\sum_{i=1}^{6} X^2$$

There are 6 values of X, each at intervals of 1 unit (for example if X_1 is 5, X_2 is 6, X_3 is 7, X_4 is 8, etc. We then add the square of each X; X_1^2 would be 25, X_2^2 would be 36, X_3^2 would be 49, etc., so we add 25 plus 36 plus 49, etc.).

Null Hypothesis and Errors

A null hypothesis is a tentatively taken position that there is no difference between two sets of values. For example, we may wonder if a given treatment lowers the blood pressure, so we compare two groups of patients, only one of which receives the treatment. The null hypothesis states that there is no effect. No other hypothesis permits us to calculate the probability that an effect has occurred. If the data examined indicate only a very small probability that the null hypothesis is true, we reject the hypothesis. There are two types of errors we may make in this connection. *Type 1 (alpha) error:* The null hypothesis is rejected when in fact it is true. *Type 2 (beta) error:* The null hypothesis is accepted when in fact it is false.

Statements concerning probability after utilization of the null hypothesis must be carefully worded. If two means are compared and a significant difference by *t* test (see later) is found, the report should indicate that if the two populations were really equal, p is the probability that such a significant *t* value would occur [1]. This is not the same as saying that p is the probability of the investigator's being correct.

Correlation

If two variables are measured for individuals in a single sample, the relationship of these variables can be studied in two ways.

CORRELATION PROBLEM. Both variables are measured as they occur spontaneously; the degree to which they relate is found. For example, we do blood counts on a series of persons and study the relation of the leukocyte count to the erythrocyte count. We might find no correlation, a positive correlation (high WBC accompanies high RBC), or a negative correlation (high WBC accompanies low RBC). The coefficient of correlation is expressed as a figure on a scale going from 1.0 to −1.0: perfect positive correlation would be 1.0, perfect negative correlation would be −1.0, no correlation would be 0.

REGRESSION PROBLEM. One variable is fixed; the other is measured to find its dispersion. For example, to each patient we give doses of 1, 2, and 3 mg. daily of a drug to lower blood pressure; we measure the lowering of blood pressure for each person following each dose. We might conclude that there was a lowering proportionate to the dose, or that there was not.

t Test

The *t* test is used to ascertain whether the means of two samples differ significantly. Example: We find that the mean height of 20 five-year-old boys is 40 inches and of 18 five-year-old girls is 37 inches. Can we accurately conclude that the boys are taller in this group, or could the difference be due to chance?

F *Test*

The *F* test determines whether the dispersions of two samples about the mean are significantly different. Example: One chemical method for measuring blood glucose has a standard deviation of 5 mg. at the 100 mg. level; another has a standard deviation of 8 mg. at the same level. Are these significantly different?

Chi-square Test

The chi-square (χ^2) test is a test for the homogeneity of populations in which values are reported as positive or negative instead of being reported numerically. Example: In a group of 50 men, 10 have gout; in a group of 60 women, 2 have gout. Does this indicate that gout is primarily a disease of men, or could the sex difference be due to chance alone?

Degrees of Freedom

Degrees of freedom (df, sometimes DF) is defined as the number of ways in which a group of numbers can vary independently. This is not an easy concept to define, to explain, or to understand. For example, we take 20 measurements of hemoglobin levels. The series has 20 degrees of freedom because no single measurement affected the other 19. However, if we calculate the mean ($\bar{x}$) of the 20 values, the series now has $n - 1$ df, or 19 df, because the twentieth value in the series cannot be changed without altering the mean.

Random Numbers

Experimental statistics relies almost entirely on a randomization of all uncontrollable variables except the one under study. Randomization is best achieved through the use of a table of random numbers that has been carefully drawn up (Appendix Table 1). Example: We wish to test the effect of a new antibiotic on significant urinary tract infection. How do we select which patients are to receive the new drug in a double-blind experiment with avoidance of bias due to age, sex, race, and other variables? We define significant urinary tract infection, then we assign each afflicted patient a serial number starting at 1 and ascending by 1's; for each of these numbers we have previously picked a corresponding random number. Patients with an odd random number, let us say, receive the drug; those with an even random number receive the placebo.

Outliers

Outliers or deviant values are figures that are obviously from a different population than those from the rest of the sample. Their identification and elimination are difficult, but necessary; their inclusion distorts the analysis of the whole sample. Example: We have 10 calcium analyses of a specimen of blood; 9 are between 8 and 9 mg., but the tenth is recorded as 87 mg. If we include it we change the mean from 8.5 to 16.3, and the *s* from .155 to 7.80! There are various formulas for identifying and eliminating outliers; none is completely satisfactory.

Bias

Bias is the term used for a difference between the true mean of a population and the mean calculated from a series of measurements. A large bias may indicate a flaw in the selection of the sample. The term encompasses conscious selection in the usual social sense but also includes inadvertent selection—it is not used in a pejorative sense in statistical jargon. Bias is also used to mean the difference between means when the true value is unknown.

Accuracy

Accuracy is closeness to the true value. In the biological material with which we deal in the clinical laboratory, we cannot know the true value. For many substances the obtained value is method dependent; this is particularly true for enzymes and protein fractions. Some substances exist in different forms which may be bound to other substances or free from them; the binding may be broken by some methods of analysis but not by others. Because we never know the absolute values, we assume that the average value for a number of laboratories using the same method is the true value until new information disproves this hypothesis.

Precision

Precision is the closeness of the results of repeated analyses performed on the same material. Precision is expressed in such terms as standard deviation, coefficient of variation, or standard error. The conditions of analysis must be specified, including method, instrumentation, reagents, whether one or more analysts were involved, and the time during which analyses were performed, i.e., day to day, within run, etc.

Nonparametric Statistics

Nonparametric statistics are statistics that do not depend on any assumption about a normal or other defined distribution of groups of numbers. They include such tests as the sign test, the signed-rank test, runs, and rank-sum. Example: We wish to compare a group of runners to decide which ones should be on the track team. We rank their performance in a series of trial runs, not on their actual time but on their competitive rank. We assign the winner in each race the rank 1, the next one rank 2, and so on. We then add the rank numbers for each runner for all the races and get a rank-sum number. In a sign test a determination is made as to how many values carry a plus sign and how many a minus sign, relative to some reference point. Example: We determine the mean value for a quality control pool to be 10. For the next eight days the analytic results always exceed 10. Can we conclude that some systematic error has developed?

In evaluating the meaning of results of these nonparametric tests we may use chi-square or percentile calculations, both illustrated elsewhere in this volume. For rank-sum tests there are good tables available (see Wilcoxon, Katti, and

Wilcox, Annotated General Bibliography). For further details on the use of these tests the reader is referred to such standard texts as Dixon and Massey (Annotated General Bibliography).

Reference

1. Youden, W. J. How to pick a winner. *Industrial and Engineering Chemistry* 50:81A (June), 1958.

2 Arithmetical Considerations

Because statistics frequently deals with a series of individual measurements, it is necessary to agree on a set of rules for handling them. A brief account of these rules and principles follows.

Individual Measurements

The value for an individual measurement depends on the accuracy with which the measurement can be made; this in turn depends on the constancy of the object to be measured and on the available instrumentation. In the medical field there are very few measurements accurate beyond three places. Furthermore, because we are interested in biological characteristics which vary considerably from person to person and in the same person from time to time, there is usually no worth to more accurate measurement. The general rule is that each figure we report implies doubt about the significance of the next figure to the right (Table 2-1).

This approach is arbitrary and involves présumptions about the accuracy of the manipulations and instrumentation. Once statistical data are available for a series of measurements, the standard deviation provides a more reliable guide. Generally speaking, the implied accuracy for an individual measurement should not exceed $s/4$. Referring to the glucose measurement in Table 2-1, assume that $s = 5$ mg., a commonly achieved figure. The report should not be read closer than 5 mg./4 or 1.25 mg. In other words, readings to about 1 mg. are reasonable and readings to 0.1 mg. would be meaningless no matter how closely one could read the photometer scale.

The temptation to report figures beyond the significant ones occurs most often in the clinical laboratory. Example: A calculation for blood urea nitrogen analyzed spectrophotometrically is 50/3.0. Should we report this as 17, 16.7, or 16.67? If we know that our spectrophotometer is accurate only to ± 2 percent, we are obviously uncertain about the third place; we believe the measured value is 16.7 ± 2 percent of 16.7, which is 16.7 ± 0.3 mg., i.e., between 16.4 and 17.0. We are unsure about the third place and are safer reporting the value as 17.

Rounding off

The principle of reporting measurements to the nearest significant figure creates the need for "rounding off." The rules for this follow:

1. If the first figure beyond the significant figure is less than 5, drop it. Example: 176.4, round off to 176.
2. If the first figure beyond the significant figure is over 5, increase the number to the left of it by one. Example: 176.6, round off to 177.

Table 2-1
Significant Figures

Measurement	Report	Number of Significant Figures	Implied Value	Implied Maximum Error
Plasma glucose	105 mg./100 ml.	3	104.5–105.5 mg.	0.5 mg
Body temperature	98.6°F	3	98.5°–98.7°F	0.1°F*
Blood pressure	165 mm. Hg	3	164.5–165.5 mm.	0.5 mm.
Serum calcium	9.2 mg./100 ml.	2	9.15–9.25 mg.	0.05 mg.

*This is an exception to the usual rule. We know that nurses read thermometers to 0.2°F; therefore our implied error is 0.1°F in the third place.

3. If the first figure beyond the significant figure is exactly 5, round off to the nearest *even* number. Examples: 175.5 to 176, 176.5 to 176.

Significant Figures in Statistical Analysis

In statistical analysis, significant figures are handled differently than are significant figures in individual measurements. If we seek the mean value of a series of measurements, each accurate to two significant places, shall we also round off the mean to two places? The answer is NO. Carry all statistical values to at least two places beyond the measured values *during* the manipulations. This is true for means, standard deviations, and similar statistics. After the final results are obtained, then it is permissible to round off if it is desirable.

For example, we study a series of blood glucose values of 101, 93, 112, and so on. We find the mean to be 102.63, the standard deviation 5.87. From these figures we plot a control chart for 95 percent confidence limits, and we plan to plot individual glucose determinations on the chart. Now we can set the middle line at 103 (not 102.63), the lower line at 91 (not 90.89), and the upper line at 114 (not 114.37). If we attempt to round off during calculations, however, we introduce substantial errors.

3 Probability

A fundamental concept in statistical thinking is that of probability, defined as the expected occurrence of an event, that is, the relative frequency with which the event is observed in a large group of trials. Conventionally, the level of significant probability is set at 19 to 1, also expressed as 95 percent, or 5 percent, or .95, or .05. Highly significant is assumed as 99 to 1, also expressed as 99 percent, or 1 percent, or .99, or .01. This may be written for a specific instance as $p < .01$, meaning that the odds are greater than 99 to 1 against the chance occurrence; or as $.05 > p > .01$, meaning that the odds exceed 19 to 1 but not 99 to 1.

There is nothing magical about these particular odds; they are arbitrary, convenient, and correspond to widely published tables. The probability chosen as significant depends on the consequences of being wrong in the context of the specific example. For example, suppose a blood test for carcinoma of the stomach yielded 5 percent false positive results in healthy individuals, so that for any single positive result $p = .05$ that the subject does not have gastric cancer. Whether this .05 level is acceptable for a useful test depends on the next procedure to be performed on the person whose test is positive. If a further harmless blood test would be the next step, then .05 is acceptable. If the next diagnostic step would be a dangerous total removal of the stomach, one would ask for much greater reliability of diagnosis than the 19 to 1 odds. To belabor the issue further, if a proposed boating expedition carried a 5 percent chance of causing sunburn as the worst hazard, most prudent people would be willing to go; if the 5 percent chance were that of being drowned, most prudent people would stay at the dock.

Most statistical tables list a number for each appropriate probability and degree of freedom. If this number is smaller than that found by experiment, the experimental value is significant at the specified level; if the number in the table is the larger, the result is not significant. Example: Appendix Table 4 gives the figure 2.776 for 4 df, 5 percent probability. Suppose that in an experiment we obtain a value of 2.630. Since this is *less* than 2.776 it is below the critical level of significance. However, because 2.630 is so close to 2.776, and because the experimental series is so small, it is wise to accumulate more data before drawing a final conclusion.

Probability as Proof

An example of an enormous controversy centering about the use of statistical probability as scientific proof is that concerning the relation between cigarette smoking and such serious ailments as lung cancer and myocardial infarcts. Those who believe that cigarettes are responsible for producing these diseases point to a very high statistical probability based on vast amounts of data that

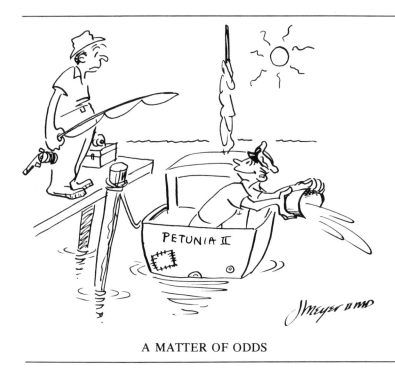

A MATTER OF ODDS

cigarette smokers suffer more frequently from these conditions and that there is some positive correlation between the number of cigarettes smoked and the disease incidence. Those who defend cigarettes criticize this type of reasoning in several ways:

1. There are many positive correlations which occur in life in which there is no known cause-and-effect relationship. High odds against the occurrence of an event do not guarantee that it will not occur. The odds against any single ticket's winning a lottery may be a million to one—but someone always wins, and the odds against his ticket were as large as those against the other 999,999.

2. There are many events which correlate to a high degree, but neither causes the other. A third factor may control both of them. The favorite example of the late Harry S. N. Greene, Professor of Pathology at Yale, went as follows: There are always many bald heads visible in the front row seats in burlesque theaters. This does not mean that going to burlesque theaters causes baldness.

We must acknowledge that high levels of probability can never be proof for a hypothesis, if we mean the kind of proof available in abstract mathematics. For practical purposes, however, we must accept the fact that all medical decision is based on considerations of probability and on picking the best odds.

Assume that a surgeon is confronted with a 16-year-old boy who has suffered for 12 hours from nausea and abdominal pain which has shifted from the epigastrium to the right lower quadrant. There is tenderness over McBurney's point, modest leukocytosis, and a normal urinalysis. The surgeon calculates that the odds greatly favor the diagnosis of acute appendicitis requiring prompt appendectomy. He is aware that there is a small chance that the illness is mesenteric adenitis, for which surgery is not helpful, and that there is a small unavoidable risk of death from surgery. The surgeon then makes his decision to operate based on what he considers to be the best odds, but he does not guarantee that he will find acute appendicitis, or that the youth might not have recovered spontaneously, or that there will not be an anesthetic or surgical mishap. Common sense is a tool equally as necessary in the use of probability statistics as in the practice of medicine.

Calculation of Probability

If we design an experiment in which only random factors are at work, we can calculate probability exactly. The classic experiments involve putting balls or discs in a box and blindly withdrawing one or more. For example, we put a black ball and a white ball in the box and remove one. The odds are 50 percent that it is white. If p = white and q = black,

$$p + q = 1 \qquad p = 0.5 \qquad \text{and} \qquad q = 0.5$$

If we repeat the experiment, the odds that each possible combination will occur are as follows (Figure 3-1):

2 white,	p^2	$= 0.25$
1 black, 1 white,	$2pq$	$= 0.50$
2 black,	q^2	$= 0.25$

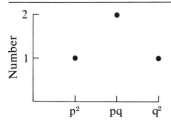

Figure 3-1
$(p + q)^2$, p = white, q = black

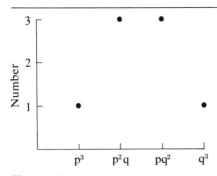

Figure 3-2
$(p + q)^3$, p = white, q = black

This is the first expansion of $(p + q)(p + q)$ or $p^2 + 2pq + q^2$. If we expand this once more by putting the ball back and picking a third time we find

$$p^3 + 3p^2q + 3pq^2 + q^3$$

with odds as follows for each combination (Figure 3-2):

3 white,	p^3	$= 0.125$
2 white, 1 black,	p^2q	$= 0.375$
1 white, 2 black,	pq^2	$= 0.375$
3 black	q^3	$= 0.125$

If we graph an infinite expansion of the experiment with a black and a white ball, we observe a curve of normal distribution (see Fig. 1-1). The total area under the curve represents all possible combinations of black and white; any segment of this area corresponds to a certain proportion of black and white.

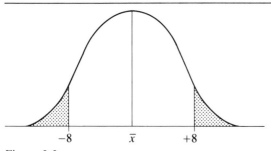

Figure 3-3
Two-tailed distribution for probability that a value will be 8 or more units *different* from the mean

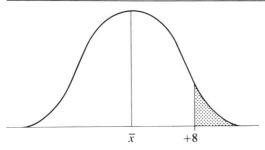

Figure 3-4
One-tailed distribution for probability that a value will be 8 or more units *higher* than the mean

The area of such a segment relative to the total area represents the odds that this particular proportion would occur by chance alone. A table is available to give mathematical odds based on multiples of $\bar{x}$ and s (see Appendix Table 6).

Probability tables may be described as one-tailed or two-tailed. If we ask, What are the odds that we will find a value 8 or more units *different* from the mean? we look to a two-sided table (Figure 3-3). If we ask, What are the odds that we will find a value 8 or more units *higher* than the mean? we look to a one-sided table (Figure 3-4). Naturally the two-sided probability for a given difference from the mean is twice that for a one-sided test; if a one-sided test result is significant at the .05 level, the same result for a two-sided test will be significant only at the .10 level.

Probability Tables

There are certain useful probability tables in the Appendix. If more comprehensive tables are desired they can be found in Fisher and Yates (Annotated General Bibliography).

TABLE 2. F DISTRIBUTION, UPPER 5 PERCENT POINTS. Used to decide whether two variances come from the same population. Values *equal to or greater than* those in the table indicate a probability of 5 percent or less, respectively, that an F value of the size observed would be obtained by chance if in fact the two variances are the same.

TABLE 3. F DISTRIBUTION, UPPER 1 PERCENT POINTS. Used to decide whether two variances come from the same population. Values *equal to or greater than* those in the table indicate a probability of 1 percent or less, respectively, that an F value of the size observed would be obtained by chance if in fact the two variances are the same.

TABLE 4. CRITICAL VALUES OF *t*. Used to calculate the probability that different means do not come from the same population. Values *higher* than those in the table indicate that populations are different.

TABLE 5. TABLES FOR TESTING SIGNIFICANCE IN 2 × 2 TABLES WITH UNEQUAL SAMPLES. Used to calculate the probability that numbers representing counts come from the same population (for series not exceeding 20 numbers in each series). For method of use see Chapter 4 and Table 4-4.

TABLE 6. CUMULATIVE NORMAL DISTRIBUTION. Used to calculate the expected percentage of the total area under a curve of normal distribution enclosed by the $\bar{x} \pm$ multiples of s.

TABLE 7. FACTORS FOR COMPUTING ONE-SIDED CONFIDENCE LIMITS FOR σ. Used to determine number of tests necessary to achieve certain confidence limits for standard deviations.

4 Normal Distribution

A series of measurements has two characteristics: (1) clustering about a central value and (2) deviation of single results from that value.

If the results are distributed in the usual random fashion they will fall into the pattern of the normal distribution curve. The arithmetic mean of all the values is the *central value*. The *deviation* is calculated in the form of the standard deviation by the formula

$$s = \sqrt{\frac{\Sigma(x - \bar{x})^2}{n - 1}}$$

where

$$s = \text{standard deviation}$$

$$\Sigma(x - \bar{x})^2 = \text{sum of } each \text{ difference from the mean squared}$$
$$n = \text{number of values entering the calculations}$$

Example: We measure the glucose value of a stable serum sample 10 times; we wish to find the mean and the standard deviation. We tabulate as shown in Table 4-1. We then calculate as follows:

$$s = \sqrt{\frac{\Sigma(x - \bar{x})^2}{n - 1}} = \sqrt{\frac{197.60}{9}} = \sqrt{21.955} = 4.69$$

Table 4-1
Calculating Mean and Standard Deviation Serum Glucose (mg./100 ml.)

Test No.	Value	$(x - \bar{x})$	$(x - \bar{x})^2$
1	48	2.2	4.84
2	39	6.8	46.24
3	47	1.2	1.44
4	50	4.2	17.64
5	39	6.8	46.24
6	50	4.2	17.64
7	49	3.2	10.24
8	51	5.2	27.04
9	41	4.8	23.04
10	44	1.8	3.24
Σ = sum	458		197.60
$\bar{x}$ = mean	45.8		
s = 4.69			

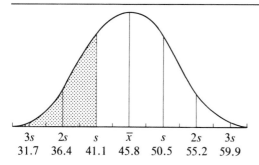

3s	2s	s	x̄	s	2s	3s
31.7	36.4	41.1	45.8	50.5	55.2	59.9

Figure 4-1
Normal distribution curve. $\bar{x} = 45.8$; $s = 4.7$. Shaded area under curve indicates area of cumulative distribution from 0 to $(\bar{x} - s) = .1587$ of total area. Glucose values 0 to 41.1 mg./100 ml.

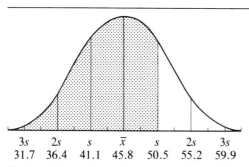

3s	2s	s	x̄	s	2s	3s
31.7	36.4	41.1	45.8	50.5	55.2	59.9

Figure 4-2
Normal distribution curve. $\bar{x} = 45.8$; $s = 4.7$. Shaded area under curve indicates area of cumulative distribution from 0 to $(\bar{x} + s) = .8413$ of total area. Glucose values 0 to 50.5 mg./100 ml.

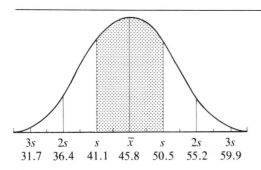

3s	2s	s	x̄	s	2s	3s
31.7	36.4	41.1	45.8	50.5	55.2	59.9

Figure 4-3
Normal distribution curve. $\bar{x} = 45.8$; $s = 4.7$. Shaded area under curve indicates area included in $\bar{x} \pm s = .6827$ of total area. Glucose values 41.1 to 50.5 mg./100 ml.

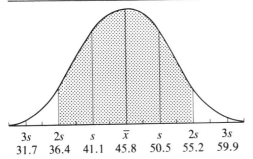

3s	2s	s	$\bar{x}$	s	2s	3s
31.7	36.4	41.1	45.8	50.5	55.2	59.9

Figure 4-4
Normal distribution curve. $\bar{x} = 45.8$; $s = 4.7$. Shaded area under curve indicates area included in $\bar{x} \pm 2s = .9545$ of total area. Glucose values 36.4 to 55.2 mg./100 ml.

The great value of the standard deviation as a measure of dispersion is that the area under the normal distribution curve can be well characterized by multiples of the standard deviation. The areas in Figures 4-1–4-5 are taken from a more complete table (see Appendix Table 6) and are related to the glucose calculations just described.

Inasmuch as we have drawn considerable conclusions as to the normal distribution from a small number of tests (only 10 in our example) we must be concerned whether this is a fair representation of the infinite population from which the tests were selected.

First we ask about the validity of the mean, 45.8. Is the true mean perhaps 47 or even 50? The diagrams in Figures 4-6 and 4-7 pose the same question schematically, assuming the same s.

The question of the significance of a difference between the observed mean and the true mean is answered through the use of the t test, the formula of which varies slightly depending on the context of the question. In the present problem we use the paired t formula

$$t = \frac{|\bar{x} - K| \sqrt{n}}{s}$$

where $\bar{x}$ = mean for the method
K = true value
n = number of tests for the method
s = standard deviation for the method
$| \; |$ = numerical difference between the enclosed symbols (therefore always a positive number)*

*If the difference is not enclosed between bars $| \; |$ there may be a negative value for t, i.e., -2.63. This result is not useful for our purposes and requires a different type of table than our Appendix Table 4.

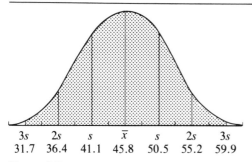

Figure 4-5
Normal distribution curve. $\bar{x}$ = 45.8; s = 4.7. Shaded area under curve indicates area included in $\bar{x} \pm 3s$ = .9973 of total area. Glucose values 31.7 to 59.9 mg./100 ml.

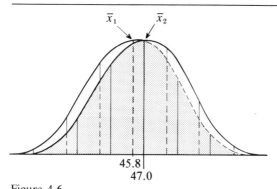

Figure 4-6
Overlapping normal distribution curves. $\bar{x}$ of one is 47.0, of other is 45.8; s of each is 1.57. Shaded area indicates values falling within both curves and is large.

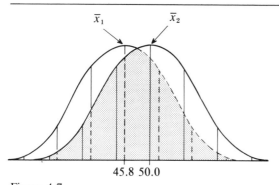

Figure 4-7
Overlapping normal distribution curves. $\bar{x}$ of one is 50.0, of other is 45.8; s of each is 1.57. Shaded area indicates values falling within both curves and is much smaller than in Fig. 4-6.

For 45.8 versus 47.0 our formula is

$$t = \frac{|\ 45.8 - 47.0\ |\ \sqrt{10}}{4.69} = \frac{1.2 \times 3.1623}{4.69} = \frac{3.7948}{4.69}$$

$$= 0.81$$

and for 45.8 versus 50.00 the formula is

$$t = \frac{|\ 45.8 - 50.0\ |\ \sqrt{10}}{4.69} = \frac{4.2 \times 3.1623}{4.69} = \frac{13.2816}{4.69}$$

$$= 2.83$$

We now look in Appendix Table 4. For 9 df we find critical values of 2.262 at the 5 percent level and 3.250 at the 1 percent level. The value of 0.81 we found in the first comparison is obviously below the critical level. The value of 2.83 in the second comparison exceeds 2.262 but not 3.250. We can therefore reject the null hypothesis that the means of 45.8 and 50.0 are from the same population beyond the 5 percent probability level.

At this point it is worth noting that the Fisher type of t table we are using is two-tailed, that is, it gives the odds that the two means are different regardless of which is larger. Some other tables are one-tailed, giving the odds that one mean is larger than the other; these use $t_{.975}$ to signify what $t_{.95}$ signifies in two-tailed tables. The subscripts refer to the probability level at which t is calculated.

A more general formula for the t test is used when two unpaired series, each of a finite number, are compared. It is applicable even when the series have different numbers and standard deviations. This formula is

$$t = \frac{|\ \bar{x}_A - \bar{x}_B\ |}{\sqrt{\left[\dfrac{(N_A - 1)s_A^2 + (N_B - 1)s_B^2}{N_A + N_B - 2} \right] \left[\dfrac{1}{N_A} + \dfrac{1}{N_B} \right]}}$$

where $\bar{x}_A$ = mean of series A
$\bar{x}_B$ = mean of series B
N_A = number of values in series A
N_B = number of values in series B
s_A^2 = variance of series A
s_B^2 = variance of series B

Example: We compare two glucose methods by repeated testing of aliquots of the same material. Method A is tried 10 times; $\bar{x} = 131.0$, $s = 21.36$. Method B is tried 20 times; $\bar{x} = 169.9$; $s = 16.01$. Substituting in the formula

$$t = \frac{\mid 131.0 - 169.9 \mid}{\sqrt{\left[\dfrac{(9 \times 456.25) + (19 \times 256.32)}{10 + 20 - 2}\right]\left[\dfrac{1}{10} + \dfrac{1}{20}\right]}}$$

$$= \frac{38.9}{\sqrt{\left[\dfrac{4106.25 + 4870.08}{28}\right] \times \dfrac{3}{20}}}$$

$$= \frac{38.9}{\sqrt{\dfrac{8976.33}{28} \times \dfrac{3}{20}}} = \frac{38.9}{\sqrt{\dfrac{26928.99}{560}}}$$

$$= \frac{38.9}{\sqrt{48.09}} = \frac{38.9}{6.935}$$

$$= 5.61$$

Looking in a t table we find that for 28 df, 5.61 is significantly beyond 1 percent, so we can conclude that the means are markedly different.

As a general rule if 10 or more tests are done in each series, a t value exceeding 2.0 is significant.

A mean value for a series of tests is more likely to approach the true value than is any one single test. The dispersion of means is therefore smaller than the dispersion of single values and is expressed as standard error (SE). The formula for this is

$$SE = \frac{\text{standard deviation}}{\sqrt{n}}$$

for n observations.

Example: Using our Table 4-1 glucose data, where s was 4.69, n was 10,

$$SE = \frac{4.69}{\sqrt{10}} = 1.48$$

This tells us that 68% of means of 10 tests would fall within 1.48 mg. of 45.8 mg. In Figure 4-8 the inner shaded area indicates the distribution of the *means* for series of 10 analyses and the outer curve indicates the distribution of values for *single analyses*.

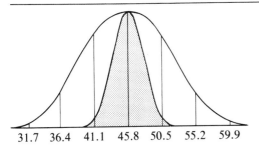

31.7 36.4 41.1 45.8 50.5 55.2 59.9

Figure 4-8
Normal distribution curve for the standard *error* of 10 analyses ($\bar{x}$ = 45.8, SE = 1.5) is shaded. Outer curve illustrates standard *deviation* of 10 analyses ($\bar{x}$ = 45.8, s = 4.7).

Next we inquire whether the dispersion (standard deviation) about the mean is likely to be representative of an infinite population. This can be answered by use of the F test whose formula is

$$F = \frac{s^2A}{s^2B}$$

where s^2A = variance of one set of values
s^2B = variance of another set

Generally s^2B is the accepted variance and s^2A the one we are studying, so that any time s^2A is smaller, the F value is less than 1, indicating that the test value (s^2A) is *not* larger than the accepted value. F values are listed in tables by df (see Appendix Tables 2 and 3).

The problem we raise in our example is this: Our s for 10 tests (9 df) is 4.6856. How small could our infinite population s be (∞ df) at the 5 percent confidence level? Substituting in the formula we find that for 9 df numerator, ∞ df denominator, the significant F figure is 1.88, therefore

$$1.88 = \frac{(4.6856)^2}{s^2B} = \frac{21.955}{s^2B}; \qquad 1.88s^2B = 21.955$$

$$s^2B = 11.678 \qquad sB = 3.417$$

so that the true sB is 3.417 or larger. We can reverse the procedure to find the largest value for sB likely at the 95 percent level by reversing the formula:

$$F = \frac{s^2B}{s^2A}$$

∞ df is now used for the numerator and 9 df for the denominator. The significant F value is 2.71 and the formula becomes

$$2.71 = \frac{s^2B}{(4.6856)^2} = \frac{s^2B}{21.955}$$

and

$$s^2B = 2.71 \times 21.955 = 59.498 \qquad sB = 7.714$$

We can now say that the odds are 19 to 1 that the true sB falls between 7.714 and 3.417.

Suppose it is found that the s of two sets of values such as sA and sB differs by more than the allowed amount—for example, that sA is 4.6856 but sB is only 1.0. We could not perform a t test of the means as described earlier, because the dispersion of sA would be so great, relative to sB, that one could conclude that the two populations were different, therefore not comparable.

Chi-square

A common problem in medical statistics is one in the following form: 50 patients are treated with medicine A and 48 with medicine B. 20 of the A's improve and 40 of the B's improve. Could this be due to chance alone? We set this up as a table:

a	b	$a + b$
c	d	$c + d$
$a + c$	$b + d$	n

where a = number of A patients who improve
b = number of B patients who improve
c = number of A's who do not improve
d = number of B's who do not improve
$a + c$ = total number A patients
$b + d$ = total number B patients
n = total number of all patients

Observed

20	40	60
30	8	38
50	48	98

Expected

30.6	29.4	60
19.4	18.6	38
50	48	98

Difference

+10.6	−10.6	0
−10.6	+10.6	0
0	0	0

Expected values were calculated by assuming that the same proportion of patients treated with A as with B should improve. Therefore if 60 of 98 patients improve, then to satisfy the null hypothesis 60/98 of each group (boxes a and b) should improve, and 38/98 of each group (boxes c and d) should not improve. The differences between the observed and the expected values for each box are listed in the table "Difference." Note that the number in boxes a, b, c, and d is the same, illustrating why chi-square (designated χ^2) has only 1 df for a comparison of two alternatives.

The chi-square figure itself is calculated as follows:

1. Square the difference for box a: $10.6^2 = 112.36$.
2. Divide by the expected value for box a: $112.36 \div 30.6 = 3.672$.
3. Do the same for b (3.822), c (5.792), and d (6.041).
4. Add these 4 values: 19.327. This is chi-square.

For most purposes it is desirable to use Yates's correction. The formula then is:

$$\chi^2 = \frac{n\left(\mid ad - bc \mid - \frac{n}{2}\right)^2}{(a + b)(c + d)(a + c)(b + d)}$$

$\mid - \mid$ means difference between, regardless of sign (therefore always a positive number).

For 1 df which we describe here (improved versus not improved, i.e., two variables, therefore 1 df), we use the following figures to assay the significant level of chi-square results:

Table 4-2
Chi-square Table for 2 df

For percentile:	95.0	97.5	99.0	99.5
Significant value is:	3.84	5.02	6.63	7.88

Values exceeding those listed are significant at the percentile level indicated. In our present example

$$\chi^2 = \frac{98(\mid 160 - 1200 \mid - 49)^2}{60 \times 38 \times 50 \times 48}$$

$$= \frac{98(991^2)}{5,472,000}$$

$$= \frac{96,243,938}{5,472,000}$$

$$= 17.59$$

This considerably exceeds our 99.5 percent percentile value of 7.88, so the odds are very large that medicine B is really better than medicine A.

Chi-square may also be used for more than two variables. For example, we can test agreement in white cell differential counts done by two different observers. Technologist A counts a smear and Job Applicant B counts the same smear. Here are the results:

	A	B
Neutrophils	62	59
Stab cells	3	12
Lymphocytes	22	25
Monocytes	9	2
Eosinophils	3	2
Basophils	1	0

The following chi-square formula is suitable for more than two variables; it omits the Yates correction:

$$\chi^2 = \sum^n \frac{(a - b)^2}{a + b}$$

where n = number of variables
a = expected value (figures from column A above)
b = observed value (figures from column B above)

We apply this to the above differential count data as follows:

	$a - b$	$(a - b)^2$	$a + b$	$\dfrac{(a - b)^2}{a + b}$
Neutrophils	3	9	121	.074
Stab cells	−9	81	15	5.40
Lymphocytes	−3	9	47	.19
Monocytes	7	49	11	4.45
Eosinophils	1	1	5	.20
Basophils	1	1	1	1.00
			$\chi^2 = \Sigma =$	11.314

We then use Table 4-3 to decide the significance of this 11.314 chi-square value.

We find that our value exceeds 11.07; therefore, it appears that the two technologists did count differently. Inspection leads us to suspect that Job Applicant B is confusing monocytes and stab cells. If we pool the stabs and monocytes to validate this hypothesis, recalculation gives a χ^2 of 1.54, much

Table 4-3
Significant Chi-square for Varying df, 95% Level

df	1	2	3	4	5	6	7	8	9	10
χ^2	3.84	5.99	7.81	9.49	11.07	12.59	14.07	15.51	16.92	18.31

less than the significant value of 9.49 for 4 df. This confirms our suspicion as to the nature of the difference.

When any series contains less than 40 individuals it is best to use a 2×2 contingency table for unequal samples (see Appendix Table 5). Such a table is somewhat confusing to use, so a sample section (Table 4-4) and description are provided.

Here we are comparing two series in which n_1 has 5 components and n_2, as indicated in the second column, has 5 or less. The question we ask is this: If we compare two similar small series and we find that series n_1 with 5 members contains a_1 positive for a certain event, how many in a second series of 5 or less (n_2) would have to be positive (a_2) for the result to be significantly different? For example, if we treated 5 patients with common colds with medicine A and 4 were cured immediately, in a second series of 4 patients with common colds, how many cures would we expect with medicine B if it were of no value?

Checking our sample section (Table 4-4) we look under $n_1 = 5, n_2 = 4, a_1 = 4$ (line underlined), and under 0.05 (0.10) we find the figures **0** .040. The boldface **0** indicates that an a_2 of zero—that is, *no* cures in 4 patients—is significantly *smaller* than 4 cures in 5 patients at a significance level of 0.10; and that it is significantly *different* from 4 in 5 at a level of .05; and that the exact probability of a_2 being equal to or less than 0 is .040. If medicine A produced 5 cures, then medicine B would be significantly less effective if it gave 1 cure or less in 4

Table 4-4
Section of 2×2 Table for Unequal Samples (from Appendix Table 5)

			Significance Level			
		a_1	0.05 (0.10)	0.025 (0.05)	0.01 (0.02)	0.005 (0.01)
$n_1 = 5$	$n_2 = 5$	5	1 .024	1 .024	**0** .004	**0** .004
		4	**0** .024	**0** .024	—	—
	4	5	1 .048	**0** .008	**0** .008	—
		4	**0** .040	—	—	—
	3	5	**0** .018	**0** .018	—	—
	2	5	**0** .048	—	—	—

Source: M. G. Natrella, *Experimental Statistics*. National Bureau of Standards Handbook 91 (Washington, D.C.: U.S. Government Printing Office, 1966, 1976).

patients at the .05 significance level and 0 cures at the 0.025 or 0.01 levels. However, even 0 cures in 4 patients would not be significant at the 0.005 level. In this context the meaning of one- and two-tailed is as follows: One-tailed, is a_1 *larger* than a_2? Two-tailed, is a_1 *different* from a_2?

It also follows in this type of table that values for a_2 exceeding the boldface values have not been shown to be different from a_1 in the series used. Obviously a larger or different series might yield a different result, but at least we know the odds for the occurrence of the a_2 value which we found.

In the use of this type of table negative rather than positive findings may have to be used. For example, we treat 5 leukemia patients with medicine A with no cures and 4 leukemia patients with medicine B with 2 cures. Is B better than A? We note that there is no place for $n_1 = 5$, $a_1 = 0$; so we reverse the question. We say medicine A gave 5 failures in 5 attempts, medicine B, 2 failures in 4 attempts. Now we enter the table with $n_1 = 5$, $n_2 = 4$, $a_1 = 5$. Values greater than 1 failure have no significance. This example is statistically valid, but the conclusion that B is not better than A is obvious nonsense; any medicine capable of giving 50 percent cures in a fatal disease is certainly worthy of further study. The answer lies in application of common sense and in additional trials.

Poisson Distribution

IRWIN M. WEISBROT

In contrast to the Gaussian distribution, which describes common events occurring about a mean and diminishing rapidly in frequency at the symmetrical tails, the Poisson distribution describes rare events. It is therefore suitably applied to blood cell counting, in which minute particles are randomly distributed within a very large volume of fluid, and also to differential counts, in which leukocytes are considered rare particles randomly distributed over an infinitely large surface. It is also appropriate for radioligand assays.

The typical shapes of two Poisson distributions are shown in Figure 4-9, which plots the probability of getting different percent band forms on a 100-cell differential count, given true values of 3 and 10 per 100 cells. The curves, particularly the one for 3 percent, are skewed toward the low end where they are limited by zero. Although the probability of getting a band count of 10 when the true level is 3 is less than .002, there is at least a theoretical possibility of getting even 100, therefore there is a long asymmetric tail to the right.

The formula for Poisson distribution is

$$p_x = \frac{(e^{-\lambda})(\lambda^x)}{x!}$$

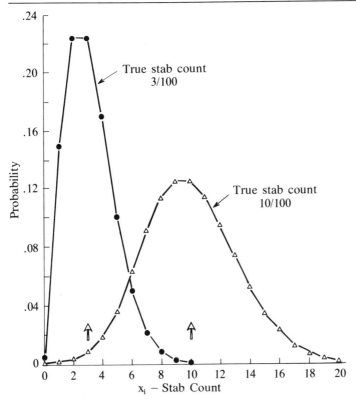

Figure 4-9

Two Poisson distributions showing the likelihood of getting various different results for the number of stab cells in a 100-cell differential count, given true values of 3 stab cells per 100 (left curve) and 10 stab cells per 100 (right curve). Note that as the true count per 100 increases the curve tends to resemble the Gaussian curve.

where in this case

p_x = probability of counting x band forms in 100 cells.

λ = true count per 100 cells.

$x!$ = "factorial," meaning the product of a descending series of whole numbers. For example 5! means $5 \times 4 \times 3 \times 2 \times 1$; 1! and 0! both = 1.

e = 2.7183, the base of the natural logarithm value in differential calculus.

This formula is easily worked on most modern desk-top programmable computers but is tedious for hand calculations. Table 4-5 will help when the numbers are small.

Table 4-5
Exponentials and Factorials

Negative exponents of e	Factorials
e^{-0} = 1.00000	0! = 1.00000000
e^{-1} = 0.36788	1! = 1.00000000
e^{-2} = 0.13533	2! = 2.00000000
e^{-3} = 0.04979	3! = 6.00000000
e^{-4} = 0.018316	4! = 24.0000000
e^{-5} = 0.006738	5! = 120.000000
e^{-6} = 0.002479	6! = 720.000000
e^{-7} = 0.000912	7! = 5,040.00000
e^{-8} = 0.000335	8! = 40,320.0000
e^{-9} = 0.000123	9! = 362,880.000
e^{-10} = 0.000045	10! = 3,628,900.00
e^{-11} = 0.000017	11! = 39,916,800.0
e^{-12} = 0.000006	12! = 479,001,600

If the true band count is 5 leukocytes per 100 cells, what is the probability that a count of 2 per 100 might occur?

$$p_x = \frac{(2.7183^{-5})(5^2)}{2!} = \frac{.00674 \times 25}{2 \times 1} = .084.$$

The probability is thus 8.4 percent. If we asked the possibility of getting a count of 2 or less, we would add the probability of counting 2 per 100, 1 per 100, and 0 per 100; the final answer would be approximately 12.5 percent.

The best way to diminish the probability of finding a count different from the true count is to classify more cells. For example, if we counted 200 cells and the true value were 10 per 200, then the probability of finding 4 per 200 is 1.9%, as determined by using the formula and entering the x and λ values for 200 cells. In practice deviations from the Poisson distribution can be expected, because the spreading of the cells is not entirely random.

As we enumerate the common cells such as neutrophils and lymphocytes, or in fact any cell whose true value is over 10 percent, the curve becomes quite Gaussian and we can use the formula $s = \sqrt{\dfrac{pq}{n}}$ (see page 65) rather than the more complex Poisson calculation.

A very important property of the Poisson distribution is that s is equal to the square root of the mean.

$$s = \sqrt{\bar{x}}$$

So if the raw count of WBC in a chamber is 200, $s = \sqrt{200} = 14.1$. Thus the

95 percent confidence interval for repeated counts, due to the randomness of the particles floating in the fluid, would be 200 ± 28. If we multiply by 50, as in the usual chamber count, the 95 percent confidence limits will be 8,600 to 11,400 with a CV of 7 percent. If we count the same sample in an electronic particle counter which actually enumerates 10,000 cells, $s = 100$ and the limits will be 9,800 to 10,200 with a CV of 1 percent. Obviously the precision of chamber counting can be improved by counting more cells.

One of the problems with chamber counts is that technologists tend to equalize counts in adjacent squares (see page 116). To test for this "equalization," have the technologist record counts for 5 tertiary squares on each side of a chamber (10 squares in all). Find the mean and then determine s by the usual formula

$$s = \sqrt{\frac{\Sigma(x - \bar{x})^2}{n - 1}}$$

Compare this actual s to that predicted by Poisson as $\sqrt{\bar{x}}$. If s is much less than $\sqrt{\bar{x}}$ there has been "equalization" because

$$\frac{s}{\sqrt{\bar{x}}}$$

is ordinarily close to 1.

In an actual experiment of this kind the 10 values obtained were 46, 60, 42, 55, 43, 44, 52, 40, 58, 49. This gave a mean of 48.9 ($\sqrt{\bar{x}} = 6.99$) and an s of 7.05. Since $\sqrt{\bar{x}}$ and s were almost identical there was no evidence of unconscious equalization or nonrandom cell distribution.

Nonnormal Distribution

Laboratory analyses themselves, as exemplified in evaluation of methods, quality control programs, or proficiency surveys, usually follow a normal distribution and lend themselves well to calculations of standard deviation and analysis of variance. However, distributions of values in human populations, normal or otherwise, may be distinctly nonnormal [2]. They may be log normal or biphasic or have some other form. Obviously such distributions are not as appropriately studied in the same way, even though standard deviation is a "robust" statistical tool. Alternative methods of establishing ranges for groups, such as calculations of log normal or percentiles, are given in Chapter 9.

Use of Median Values

Median values are appropriately used when the data are so mixed that a true picture is not given by the arithmetic mean. A commonly used example is that of "average" annual income: 4 families earn $10,000, 10 families earn $12,000,

4 families earn $15,000, and 1 family earns $1,000,000. The "average" (arithmetic mean) is $64,211, but none of the families is anywhere close to this figure. On the other hand, the median (fiftieth percentile or P50) value of $12,000 describes the income for an average family in this group quite accurately.

We used this type of calculation when studying how many minutes it took for reports to get from the laboratory to the Emergency Department [1]. For 26 instances the numerical distribution was:

Minutes elapsed	Number of instances
0	4
4	1
5	8
6	1
8	1
10	4
15	3
16	1
20	1
30	2

The arithmetical mean of this group is 9.2 minutes; the median (P50) is 5 minutes. The true picture is given by the range (0–30) and the median (5). This discrepancy between mean and median was more marked when we followed reports to the nursing units; some were received promptly, but a few were a week in transit and would have greatly increased the "average" time.

An inappropriate way of using median values is employed at the Center for Disease Control in evaluating chemistry survey results [3]. "A second parameter, clinical requirements, is established as the reference laboratory median plus or minus ¼ of the normal range." If the mean and median are the same this is satisfactory, but there is no reason to use the median. If they differ, the concept of setting Gaussian limits about a non-Gaussian central value is incorrect.

References

1. Barnett, R. N., Bimmel, M., Peracca, M., and Roseman, K. Time intervals between ordering and obtaining laboratory test results. *Lab Med* 7:18–21; 34, 1976.
2. Elveback, L. R., Guillier, C. L., and Keating, F. R. Health, normality and the ghost of Gauss. *J.A.M.A.* 211:69–75, 1970.
3. Proficiency testing summary analysis: Clinical chemistry 1975, IV. Atlanta: Center for Disease Control, 1976.

5 Analysis of Variance

We have already said that variance (s^2) has an advantage as a statistic over standard deviation (s) in that one can add, subtract, and otherwise manipulate s^2, and one cannot do this with s. For example, we have made three sets of five measurements each and determined the s for each set as 1, 2, and 2.5, respectively. If we wish to determine s for the three series taken together we should *not* add 1, 2, and 2.5 to get 5.5, then divide by 3 to get an s of 1.83. Instead we convert to variance by squaring each s, yielding 1, 4, and 6.25; add these to give 11.25; divide the summed variances by 3 to yield 3.75; and take the square root, giving 1.94 as the pooled s.

We also make use of a mathematical trick for calculating variances from a series of numbers. The usual method requires the following manipulations:

1. List the numbers.
2. Add them. $\qquad\qquad\qquad\qquad\qquad\qquad\qquad \Sigma x$
3. Divide by n to get mean $\bar{x}$. $\qquad\qquad\qquad\qquad \dfrac{\Sigma x}{n} = \bar{x}$
4. Subtract $\bar{x}$ from each number to obtain differences. $\qquad\qquad\qquad\qquad\qquad x - \bar{x} = d$
5. Square each difference. $\qquad\qquad\qquad\qquad (x - \bar{x})^2 = d^2$
6. Add squares to get sum of squares. $\qquad\qquad\qquad \Sigma d^2$
7. Divide by $n - 1$ to get s^2. $\qquad\qquad\qquad \dfrac{\Sigma d^2}{n - 1} = s^2$

Example: 1 sample, 4 glucose estimations as given in Table 5-1.

A better method for more general use is as follows (Table 5-2):

1. List the numbers.
2. Add them. $\qquad\qquad\qquad\qquad\qquad\qquad\qquad \Sigma x$
3. Square this sum and divide by n. This sum squared and divided by n is a correction factor which will later be subtracted from the sum of the squares of the sample values. $\qquad\qquad \dfrac{(\Sigma x)^2}{n}$
4. Square each number. Add the squares. $\qquad\qquad \Sigma x^2$
5. Subtract the correction factor (3) from the sum of the squares (4). This is the difference in the sums of the squares. $\qquad\qquad \Sigma x^2 - \dfrac{(\Sigma x)^2}{n}$
6. Divide by $n - 1$ to get the variance (s^2). $\qquad \dfrac{\Sigma x^2 - \dfrac{(\Sigma x)^2}{n}}{n - 1}$

Table 5-1
Calculating Mean and Standard Deviation(s) of Glucose (mg./100 ml.)
First Method

Value	d from 98	d^2
96	2	4
99	1	1
94	4	16
103	5	25
$\Sigma\,392$		46
$\bar{x} = 98$		
$s^2 = 46/3 = 15.3$ $\quad$ $s = 3.91$		

Table 5-2
Calculating Mean and Standard Deviation(s) of Glucose (mg./100 ml.)
Second Method

	Numbers (x)		Squares (x^2)
	96		9,216
	99		9,801
	94		8,836
	103		10,609
Sum of numbers (Σx)	392	Sum of squares (Σx^2)	38,462
Squared sum $(\Sigma x)^2$	153,664	Subtract $(\Sigma x)^2/n$	38,416
Divide by n (= 4)	38,416	Difference in sum of squares	46
$s^2 = 46$ divided by $n - 1 = 46/3 = 15.3$. $s = 3.91$.			
This is the same as the result in Table 5-1.			

The second form of calculation is more difficult manually but lends itself readily to handling by calculators, particularly the automatic ones which can simultaneously total x and x^2. There are two precautions which must be observed. First, carry out all calculations to at least three places beyond the original figures. Second, avoid arithmetical errors because they are vastly magnified during the calculations.

We can now proceed to analysis of variance utilizing the method just described for finding the difference in the sums of squares. The mathematical model is difficult only in the details of lining up the individual components.

Problem One

Using aliquots of a stable serum sample we perform a series of glucose analyses by a single method, as follows: We submit two aliquots as blind unknowns to each of two technologists on each of three different days. We assume that they will be randomly placed in each run. Our questions are:

1. What are the mean and the variance for the whole group of 12 samples?
2. What is the contribution to variance of
   a. the 2 technologists?
   b. the 2 samples in each run?
   c. the 3 days?
   d. the residual variance of the method itself?

The actual values found are shown in Table 5-3. Now calculate as shown in Table 5-4.

1. Put all the values in a row (column 1).
2. Calculate all the squares; add (column 2).
3. Add the values in column 1. Square this sum. Divide by 12. We use this as the correction factor in our further calculations.
4. Subtract from Σx^2 (item 2 above).

Now we will consider each variable, lining up the data in rows and columns. We will begin with the contribution of the technologists. The values for each technologist are listed in columns (Table 5-5).

Our next question concerns the difference between the two samples, so we line up the data for each sample (Table 5-6). Finally, we wish to study the influence of day-to-day variation, so we line up the data by days (Table 5-7).

We now prepare a table (Table 5-8). The degrees of freedom were calculated as follows. For the total 12 values, df is 1 less or 11. For the two technologists it is 1 less, or 1, and for the two samples it is 1 less, or 1. For the three days it is 1 less, or 2 degrees. Subtracting the degrees of freedom for each of the variables $(1 + 1 + 2 = 4)$ from the total df for all the values (11) leaves 7 for the remainder.

Table 5-3
ANOVA Problem One
Glucose (mg./100 ml.), Raw Data*

| Day | Technologist A | | Technologist B | |
	Sample 1	Sample 2	Sample 1	Sample 2
1	97 a	100 d	101 g	93 j
2	98 b	96 e	94 h	99 k
3	99 c	93 f	100 i	95 l

*Each value is lettered for identification in the calculations.

Table 5-4
ANOVA Problem One
Glucose (mg./100 ml.), Calculating Sums of Squares*

	Column 1 (x)		Column 2 (x^2)
	97 a		9,409
	98 b		9,604
	99 c		9,801
	100 d		10,000
	96 e		9,216
	93 f		8,649
	101 g		10,201
	94 h		8,836
	100 i		10,000
	93 j		8,649
	99 k		9,801
	95 l		9,025
Σx	1,165	Σx^2	113,191.000
$(\Sigma x)^2$	1,357,225	Subtract	113,102.083
Divide by $n = 12$	113,102.083	Difference in sums of squares	88.917

*Each value is lettered for identification in the calculations.

Table 5-5
ANOVA Problem One
Glucose (mg./100 ml.), Calculation to Compare Technologists*

	Technologist A		Technologist B
	97 a		101 g
	98 b		94 h
	99 c		100 i
	100 d		93 j
	96 e		99 k
	93 f		95 l
	Σx_A 583		Σx_B 582
	$(\Sigma x_A)^2$ 339,889		$(\Sigma x_B)^2$ 338,724
$(\Sigma x_A)^2 + (\Sigma x_B)^2$			678,613
Divide by number of rows (6)			113,102.167
Subtract total correction factor			113,102.083
Difference in sums of squares			.084

*Each value is lettered for identification in the calculations.

Table 5-6
ANOVA Problem One
Glucose (mg./100 ml.), Calculation to Compare Samples*

		Sample 1		Sample 2
		97 a		100 d
		98 b		96 e
		99 c		93 f
		101 g		93 j
		94 h		99 k
		100 i		95 l
	Σx_1	589	Σx_2	576
	$(\Sigma x_1)^2$	346,921	$(\Sigma x_2)^2$	331,776
$(\Sigma x_1)^2 + (\Sigma x_2)^2$				678,697
Divide by number of rows (6)				113,116.167
Subtract correction factor				113,102.083
Difference in sums of squares				14.084

*Each value is lettered for identification in the calculations.

Table 5-7
ANOVA Problem One
Glucose (mg./100 ml.), Calculation to Compare Days*

		Day 1	Day 2	Day 3
		97 a	98 b	99 c
		100 d	96 e	93 f
		101 g	94 h	100 i
		· 93 j	99 k	95 l
	Σx^1 391	Σx_2 387	Σx_3 387
	$(\Sigma x_1)^2$ 152,881	$(\Sigma x_2)^2$ 149,769	$(\Sigma x_3)^2$ 149,769
$(\Sigma x_1)^2 + (\Sigma x_2)^2 + (\Sigma x_3)^2$				452,419
Divide by number of rows (4)				113,104.750
Subtract correction factor				113,102.083
Difference in sums of squares				2.667

*Each value is lettered for identification in the calculations.

Table 5-8
ANOVA Problem One
Final Calculations

| Category | df | Analysis of Variance (ANOVA) | | |
		Difference in Sums of Squares*	Variance (diff/df)	F Ratio
Total	11	88.917	8.083	
Technologists	1	0.084	0.084	.01
Samples	1	14.084	14.084	1.37
Days	2	2.667	1.333	.13
Remainder	7	72.082	10.297	

*In this table the difference in sums of squares was derived from the previous calculations down to the line "remainder." Remainder is the difference between the total difference (88.917) and the sum of the known differences (0.084 + 14.084 + 2.667 = 16.835), and is therefore 72.082.

Variance is then calculated for each category by dividing the difference in sum of squares by the df for that category. Finally, the F ratio is calculated as the ratio of variance for each known category to the variance for the remainder. F values of less than 1 are never significant, so we ignore the .01 and .13 F values. To evaluate the 1.37 value for samples we enter an F table with the degrees of freedom indicated, in this case 1. We find that for 1 df in the numerator and 7 df in the denominator, the significant level at 5 percent probability is 5.59, which is much larger than our value. We decide therefore that none of the three variables tested is significant in relation to the remainder, which comprises the inherent variability of the method.

In reviewing this chapter for the first edition, the late Dr. W. J. Youden had the following comments.*

The above analysis of variance fits very well the problem at hand. It fits because we may properly assume that if there should be any change in sample value from day to day then both (or all) samples will change to the same degree. This is a fair assumption if the samples are essentially closely similar in character. Equally we may reasonably assume that, if there is a difference between the samples, there is no reason to expect this difference to depend on which technician does the work. There are situations in which such assumptions may be unjustified. For example, if two samples of quite different nature are determined by two methods that differ in principle, it may well happen that the difference found between the samples does depend on which method is used. Statisticians describe this case as one in which there is an "interaction" between samples and methods. These cases are not discussed here.

I illustrate my method of checking computations as follows. Starting at step four I run my eye down the column of x's, pick the smallest (93), and diminish every x by this amount. This "coding" of the data means one can usually write down the squares of (x − constant) from memory (Table 5-9). All the remaining computations could just as well be performed using the coded values of x with similar savings.

*Personal communication, December 29, 1969.

Table 5-9
ANOVA Problem One
"Coding" of Data

x	$x - 93$*	$(x - 93)^2$
97	4	16
98	5	25
99	6	36
100	7	49
96	3	9
93	0	0
101	8	64
94	1	1
100	7	49
93	0	0
99	6	36
95	2	4
	49	289.000

$49^2 = 2,401$ Subtract 200.083

Divide by 12 $= 200.083$ Difference in sums of squares   88.917

*Smallest value in x column (93) subtracted from each other value.

There is another check on the arithmetic. In Table 5-5 we find

	Technologist A	Technologist B
Σx	583	582

Difference in sums = 1; difference squared = 1; divide by 12 = 0.0833.

In Table 5-6 we note

	Sample 1	Sample 2
Σx	589	576

Difference in sums = 13; difference squared = 169; divide by 12 = 14.0833.

And in Table 5-7 we find

	Day 1	Day 2	Day 3
Σx	391	387	387

Difference in sums is

day 1 − day 2 = 4;   squared = 16
day 1 − day 3 = 4;   squared = 16
day 2 − day 3 = 0;   squared = 0
sum of squared difference   = 32
divide by 12   = 2.667

This simple check is not shown in statistics texts!

Table 5-10
ANOVA Problem Two
Calcium (mg./100 ml.), Raw Data

Specimen No.	Serum		Plasma	
	Sample 1	Sample 2	Sample 1	Sample 2
1	9.2	9.1	9.2	9.3
2	10.0	9.9	9.8	9.5
3	8.4	8.4	8.4	8.4
4	8.6	8.7	8.5	8.7
5	9.3	9.8	9.0	9.0
6	8.8	8.9	8.9	8.8
7	8.6	8.7	9.5	8.7
8	8.6	8.7	8.9	8.6

Table 5-11
ANOVA Problem Two
Calcium (mg./100 ml.), Comparison of Samples

	Sample 1		Sample 2
	9.2		9.1
	10.0		9.9
	8.4		8.4
	8.6		8.7
	9.3		9.8
	8.8		8.9
	8.6		8.7
	8.6		8.7
	9.2		9.3
	9.8		9.5
	8.4		8.4
	8.5		8.7
	9.0		9.0
	8.9		8.8
	9.5		8.7
	8.9		8.6
Σx_1	143.7	Σx_2	143.2
$(\Sigma x_1)^2$	20,649.69	$(\Sigma x_2)^2$	20,506.24

$(\Sigma x_1)^2 + (\Sigma x_2)^2$	41,155.930
Divide by number of rows (16)	2,572.246
Subtract correction factor	2,572.238
Difference in sums of squares	.008

Problem Two

Using the atomic absorption method for calcium analyses, we wish to determine whether the results on serum and plasma are the same or different. The technologist takes eight samples of blood, splitting each into serum and plasma. She analyzes each sample twice as blind unknowns. The results are as shown in Table 5-10.

We first calculate the totals. We add all values (286.90), square the sum (82,311.61), and divide by 32 to get a correction factor of 2,572.238. Our sum of squares of each value is 2,578.950 so the difference of the sums of squares is 6.712.

Second, we line up the samples 1 and 2 as shown in Table 5-11. Next we line up the serum and plasma values (Table 5-12). Finally, we wish to evaluate the effect of the different patient specimens, so we line the specimens up in columns as shown in Table 5-13.

Table 5-12
ANOVA Problem Two
Calcium (mg./100 ml.). Comparison of Serum and Plasma

		Serum		Plasma
		9.2		9.2
		10.0		9.8
		8.4		8.4
		8.6		8.5
		9.3		9.0
		8.8		8.9
		8.6		9.5
		8.6		8.9
		9.1		9.3
		9.9		9.5
		8.4		8.4
		8.7		8.7
		9.8		9.0
		8.9		8.8
		8.7		8.7
		8.7		8.6
	Σx_1	143.7	Σx_2	143.2
	$(\Sigma x_1)^2$	20,649.69	$(\Sigma x_2)^2$	20,506.24
$(\Sigma x_1)^2 + (\Sigma x_2)^2$				41,155.930
Divide by number of rows (16)				2,572.246
Subtract correction factor				2,572.238
Difference in sums of squares				.008

Table 5-13
ANOVA Problem Two
Calcium (mg./100 ml.). Comparison of Specimens

	Specimen No.							
	1	2	3	4	5	6	7	8
	9.2	10.0	8.4	8.6	9.3	8.8	8.6	8.6
	9.1	9.9	8.4	8.7	9.8	8.9	8.7	8.7
	9.2	9.8	8.4	8.5	9.0	8.9	9.5	8.9
	9.3	9.5	8.4	8.7	9.0	8.8	8.7	8.6
Σx	36.8	39.2	33.6	34.5	37.1	35.4	35.5	34.8
$(\Sigma x)^2$	1,354.24	1,536.64	1,128.96	1,190.25	1,376.41	1,253.16	1,260.25	1,211.04

$(\Sigma x)^2$ (the sum of the squares of the sums of columns 1–8) 10,310.95
Divide by number of rows (4)   2,577.738
Subtract correction factor   2,572.238
Difference in sums of squares   5.500

Table 5-14
ANOVA Problem Two
Final Calculations

		Analysis of Variance		
Category	df	Difference in Sums of Squares	Variance (diff/df)	F Ratio
Total	31	6.712	.216	
Samples 1 & 2	1	.008	.008	.148
Serum-plasma	1	.008	.008	.148
Patients	7	5.500	.786	14.556
Remainder	22	1.196	.054	

Our chart is then as given in Table 5-14.

The fact that the sample variance equaled the serum-plasma variance was entirely coincidental. The patient F value of 14.556 is now taken to a 5 percent F table for 7 df in the numerator and 22 df in the denominator. The table value is 2.46; our value greatly exceeds this, indicating that almost all the variation in the total experiment results from differences between patients—which we expect. We can also conclude that the difference between duplicate samples and the difference between plasma and serum are very similar and very small. The major variation due to the method is in the ''remainder,'' which is the inherent variability of the method.

6 Linear Regression

IRWIN M. WEISBROT

When Galton, a cousin of Darwin, discovered that tall parents and short parents produced children who were often not quite so tall or short, but rather tended toward the usual human stature, the idea of "regression to the mean" was born. The Victorian hope of infinitely improving the species was replaced, at least for some, by resigned acceptance of the stolid mediocrity imposed by a stable gene pool.

In this same vein, the concept that scattered data points can be characterized by an equation that describes the relationship among the points and, more importantly, allows prediction of future points, is a powerful tool that we all use intuitively. The technique of describing data to fit a straight-line equation (linear regression) is the most common regression technique used in the clinical laboratory. Regression of data to fit other curve forms can be done, but our concern in this chapter is mostly with straight lines.

Conventions Used in Linear Regression

Simply put, linear regression statistics permit an answer to the following question: If I know something about x, do I know something about y? By custom, x refers to the independent variable and y to the dependent variable. Thus, if we wanted to study how incubation time affects the absorbance of a reaction, time values would be x and absorbance values would be y. Again by convention, x values are plotted along the horizontal axis (the abscissa) and y values along the vertical axis (the ordinate). The two axes cross at the origin. See Figure 6-1.

The axes often have the same scale, so that a given distance along each axis represents the same numerical value. If the two axes are not numerically equivalent, however, be cautious about conclusions drawn by inspecting a scattergram or even a line drawn through the data points. Sometimes it is not possible to make both scales the same. For example, in a plot of units of enzyme activity versus temperature the scales are arbitrary with respect to each other; but if the data concern platelet counts by method x vs. method y we would expect the axes to be numerically equal. See Figure 6-2.

As shown in Figure 6-2, a given x and y pair produce an (x,y) point.

Scatter Plot of Data

Useful conclusions about paired data values can often be drawn by inspecting a simple data plot before performing calculations. We can often decide if it is reasonable to assume that x and y are linear or nonlinear (curved) with respect to each other, random or unrelated to each other, or even inversely related to each other. This simple expedient may be more useful than elaborate calculations. See Figure 6-3.

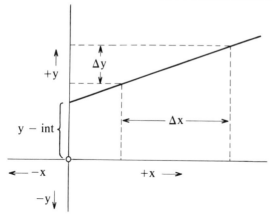

Figure 6-1
Basic format of a line with a positive slope and a positive y-intercept.

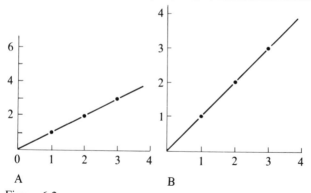

A   B

Figure 6-2
Both lines have the same slope, and in both cases, $y = x$; but in A the scales differ, the y scale being only half the graphic size of x, whereas in B the scales are equal.

The Basic Straight-Line Equation

The linear relationship is expressed by the equation

$$y = mx + b$$

where y = dependent variable
      x = independent variable
      m = slope ($\Delta y/\Delta x$), a proportionality constant which states that there is a given average change in y for a given change in x.
      b = y-intercept, the point at which the line intersects the y axis when $x = 0$.

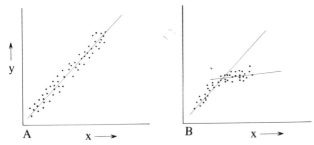

Figure 6-3
The scattergram in A appears well-represented by a single straight line. In B the data are curved, or perhaps can be described by two lines. Plotting on semi-log or log-log paper might produce a straight line.

If the line goes through the origin, then the y-intercept $= 0$ and the equation simplifies to $y = mx$. And if $\Delta y = \Delta x$, then the slope $= 1$ and the equation becomes $y = x$, a simple identity. On axes of equal numerical value the line described by this last equation would make an angle of 45 degrees and pass through the origin. Figure 6-4 shows a number of lines with their equations.

Linear Regression Methods

Graphic Methods
A simple way to determine linear parameters is to draw the best line by eye. Table 6-1 lists data for a cyanmethemoglobin calibration using dilutions of a concentrated certified standard plotted against absorbances.

A single straight line which best fits the points is shown in Figure 6-5 and goes through the origin, assuming (not always the case for all analytes) that zero concentration has zero absorbance. A convenient Δy is taken (in this case $20 - 5 = 15$), and for the same interval Δx is observed to equal $+.27$. Therefore, the slope $\Delta y/\Delta x = 15/.27 = 55.5$. The equation for y in terms of x (y on x) is then $y = 55.5x + 0$. In practical terms this means the hemoglobin concentration $= 55.5$ times the absorbance reading.

If the y-intercept were not zero, it could be determined graphically by extending the drawn line across the y-axis (where $x = 0$) and reading the y value. If it were not practical to have the x-axis extend to zero, the y-intercept could be determined from the equation

$$y = mx + b \qquad \text{or} \qquad b = y - mx$$

where b is the y-intercept

The astute reader might question if x and y were appropriately assigned, claiming that absorbancy should be y because it is related to the cyanmet-

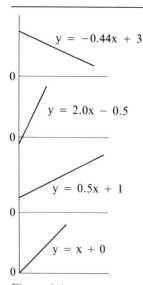

Figure 6-4
Each line is drawn on axes extending from zero. To interpret the slope, ask: for each unit x increases, how many units does y increase or decrease? As in these illustrations a decreasing y (as x increases) produces a negative slope.

hemoglobin concentrations which are calculated from an independent standard subject to many manufacturing controls. All this is true but the equation as derived is more useful to us than the opposite form would be.

While the graphic method is satisfactory for use with a few points which have little or no scatter around the estimated line, it is subject to considerable bias when used with a large scattergram. For this type of data more rigorous methods are desired.

The Group Averages Method

For large numbers of points reasonably good estimates of line parameters can be made by a simplification of the method of group averages. The (x,y) points

Table 6-1
HiCN Calibration

x Absorbance	y Hemoglobin concentration (g/dl.)
.080	4.0
.140	8.0
.215	12.0
.290	16.0
.350	20.0

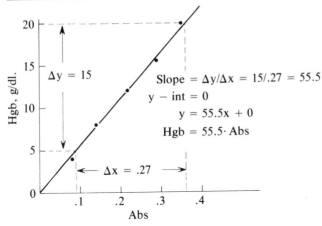

Figure 6-5
Best eye fit of HiCN calibration data.

are grouped into low, middle, and high thirds, and the average x and y values for each group are taken. Table 6-2 lists data obtained from a comparison of leukocyte counts done on two different electronic counters, x being the reference instrument and y being a new instrument under investigation.

For the present, ignore all but the x and y columns in that rather crowded table and calculate the low, middle, and high average points by making an arbitrary division into thirds, as in Table 6-3.

We have now established a low and high (x,y) from which we get Δx and Δy:

	x	y
High	10.13	10.13
Low	3.70	3.73
Δ	6.43	6.40

Then the slope $= \Delta y/\Delta x$
$$= 6.40/6.43 = 0.9953$$

If y were inversely related to x (with y values decreasing as x values increase), the slope would be a negative number.

Now that we have the slope ($m = .9953$), the y-intercept b is calculated by rearranging our equation $y = mx + b$ to solve for b, using the means ($\bar{x}$ and $\bar{y}$) shown at the bottom of the first two columns in Table 6-2.

$$b = \bar{y} - m\bar{x}$$
$$b = 6.80 - (.9953)(6.82) = 6.80 - 6.788 = +.012$$

The final solution is

$$y = .9953x + .012$$

Table 6-2
WBC by Two Electronic Cell Counters, $\times$ 10^3/mm.[3]

Test	x	y	x^2	y^2	xy	y_c	(d) $y - y_c$	$(d)^2$ $(y - y_c)^2$
1	3.1	3.2	9.61	10.24	9.92	3.184	.016	.000256
2	3.9	4.0	15.21	16.00	15.60	3.962	.038	.001444
3	4.1	4.0	16.81	16.00	16.40	4.156	−.156	.024336
4	4.5	4.8	20.25	23.04	21.60	4.545	.255	.065025
5	6.7	6.7	44.89	44.89	44.89	6.683	.017	.000289
6	7.5	7.0	56.25	49.00	52.50	7.461	−.461	.212521
7	8.0	7.9	64.00	62.41	63.20	7.947	−.047	.002209
8	9.0	9.3	81.00	86.49	83.70	8.919	.381	.145161
9	10.4	10.2	108.16	104.04	106.08	10.280	−.080	.006400
10	11.0	10.9	121.00	118.81	119.90	10.863	.037	.001369
Σ	68.2	68.0	537.18	530.92	533.79	—	.000	.459010
Averages	6.82	6.80						

which means that for any given value of x we can find the expected average value of y by multiplying the x value by .9953 and adding .012. Remember, slopes and intercepts can be either negative or positive, so watch the signs!

Note that the midpoint (x,y) average was not used, but that it can be plotted as a point on a graph. The position of this point near the line extending between the low and high points can serve as a visual guide for the goodness of fit of the line to the data. In the complete nonsimplified group averages solution, an elaborate ANOVA is done which includes the middle point data so as to yield unbiased estimates for m and b.

The Least Squares Method

The least squares method is the most commonly employed technique and the simplest one to use in programming desk-top computers. It provides the best estimates of slope and intercept. As its name implies, it positions a straight line among the points on a graph in such a way that the sum of the squares of the vertical distances from each point to the line is the smallest value possible.

For purposes of calculation and programming, set up a table like Table 6-2. In this table x and y are the actual values involved and y_c is a value of y for a given x value (x_i) calculated by means of the linear equation we are about to derive. This equation will allow us to calculate a very useful statistic, $S_{y \cdot x}$ (standard error of y in terms of x or "S sub y on x"), which is a quantitative estimate of how much the data points are dispersed around the line. This statistic is

Table 6-3
Calculating Group Averages

Group	Values	Total	Divisor	Group Average
Low x	3.1, 3.9, 4.1	11.1	3	3.70
Low y	3.2, 4.0, 4.0	11.2	3	3.73
Middle x	4.5, 6.7, 7.5, 8.0	26.7	4	6.68
Middle y	4.8, 6.7, 7.0, 7.9	26.4	4	6.60
High x	9.0, 10.4, 11.0	30.4	3	10.13
High y	9.3, 10.2, 10.9	30.4	3	10.13

sometimes called the "standard error of the estimate," a term which tends to create confusion.

If you were to program a computer to do these calculations, each column would be placed in its storage or memory. While rounding off of decimals is necessary here to make the example easier to follow, in actual practice (especially with a programmable computer) we would carry as many decimals as possible, rounding off only at the very end of the calculations.

From the sums and averages shown in Table 6-2, the slope (m) and y-intercept (b) are derived:

$$m = \frac{n\Sigma xy - (\Sigma x)(\Sigma y)}{n\Sigma x^2 - (\Sigma x)^2}$$

$$b = \bar{y} - m\bar{x}$$

Plugging in the data from Table 6-2, m and b are calculated as follows:

$$m = \frac{10(533.79) - (68.2)(68.0)}{10(537.18) - (68.2)^2} = \frac{700.3}{720.56} = +.972$$

$$b = 6.80 - (.972)(6.82) = +.171$$

and the final form of the equation for y on x is:

$$y = .972x + .171$$

You may have noted that the m and b found by the least squares method differ slightly from those derived from the same data by the group averages method. Part of the difference derives from the incompleteness of the group averages solution, part is due to early decimal rounding, and part is intrinsic to the two different methods of calculation and the assumptions underlying them.

Calculation of $S_{y \cdot x}$

We have now derived the equation of the line by two methods which give fairly similar expressions:

$y = .9953x + .012$ (Group Averages)

$y = .972x + .171$ (Least Squares)

With either of these we can answer the following question: Supposing there were no changes in the two instrument systems due to temperature, aging, calibration, etc., what value would instrument y give if reference instrument x produced a value of $x_i = 6.5 \times 10^3$ WBC per microliter?

Confining our example to the least squares equation we would predict $y_c = 6.49$, which implies very good agreement. But inspection of the individual x and y values in Table 6-2 indicates that y is sometimes higher or lower than x and suggests some intermethod variability.

$S_{y \cdot x}$ provides an estimate of the magnitude of that variability. Using the least squares solution, proceed by calculating y_c for each x_i in Table 6-2. Thus for $x_i = 3.1$, $y_c = 3.184$. (Don't round off too soon.) Next, take the differences between the actual y and y_c and list them in the appropriate column, as shown in the table. Now, anyone who has progressed this far in the book knows for certain that a statistician, given a list of differences, will square and sum almost by reflex. And, of course, the last column in Table 6-2 does just that.

Σd^2 is placed in the usual formula for standard deviation, except that the numerator is $n - 2$ rather than $n - 1$. (An extra degree of freedom is lost because y_c is a function of x.)

$$S_{y \cdot x} = \sqrt{\frac{\Sigma (y - y_c)^2}{n - 2}} = \sqrt{\frac{.45901}{8}} = .240$$

$S_{y \cdot x}$ is a standard deviation which describes the dispersion of data points around the least squares fit (or any other method of fitting the line.) Roughly, $\pm 2 S_{y \cdot x}$ comprises the 95 percent confidence interval within which our estimate $y_c = 6.49$ lies. This indicates that, based on the data we have, future single values of y could well be as low as 6.0 or as high as 7.0.

Significance of Linear Regression

Linear regression provides the clinical laboratory with two useful tools:

1. It provides a simple and general descriptive statement relating one set of observations to another in an easily visualized form.
2. It allows prediction of future values of the dependent variable.

These tools are particularly valuable in comparing methods or instruments.

Regarding the descriptive value of linear regression, the statement $y = x + 0.5$ tells us that 0.5 units must be added to the x value to predict a future y value, or that a *bias* of 0.5 exists between the x and y values. Indeed, the y-intercept concept is analogous to the concept of bias as used in t-test statistics. Pursuing this idea further, Table 6-4 demonstrates the relationships between linear and t-test statistics in detecting different types of errors between methods [3].

Observe from this table that linear regression allows bias or systematic error between methods to be dissected into two components: constant error (y-intercept) and proportional error (slope), whereas t-test statistics reveal only a single bias value which includes constant and proportional components.

Table 6-5 provides a comparison of the leukocyte counts recorded in Table 6-2 and contrasts the linear regression statistics with paired t-test statistics done on the same data.

The t-test bias predicts the future bias well only at the mean of the series, whereas they y-intercept permits estimates of errors over the entire range. Even more useful is the knowledge that there is a proportional error of -2.8 percent, so that values of y tend to be 2.8 percent lower than values of x (thence "corrected" by a constant upward error of $+.171$ which becomes less "correcting" as individual values of x depart from the mean).

Proportional errors usually imply errors in calibration (or for particle counters, errors in coincidence correction or flow volume). During our evaluations of instruments we frequently note slopes not equal to 1 which can be brought close to the reference method (slope = 1) by improved calibration techniques.

In determining confidence intervals for the future, *single* values of y, $\pm 2S_{y \cdot x}$ suffice for rough estimates, but extensive calculations which compensate for

Table 6-4
Elucidation of Errors by t-test and Linear Regression

	Type of Error		
Test	Random	Constant	Proportional
Least squares			
slope	no	no	yes
y-intercept	no	yes	no
$S_{y \cdot x}$	yes	no	no
t-test			
bias	no	yes	yes
s_d*	yes	no	yes
r†	yes	no	no

*Standard deviation of differences.
†Correlation coefficient.
Source: Modified from Westgard and Hunt [3] by permission.

Table 6-5
t-test Versus Linear Regression Statistics for WBC Instrument Comparison, Using Data
from Table 6-2

t-test		Linear Regression	
$\bar{x}$	6.82	$\bar{x}$	6.82
$\bar{y}$	6.80	$\bar{y}$	6.80
bias	.020	y-intercept	.171
s_d	.240	proportional error*	−2.8%
		$S_{y \cdot x}$	.240

*Calculated as slope by least squares minus 1, or .972 minus 1, times 100.

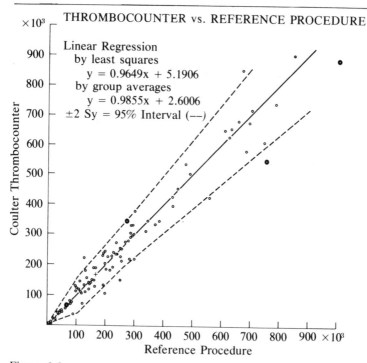

Figure 6-6
± $2S_{y \cdot x}$ envelope. Platelet counts by chamber reference method (x) vs. an electronic
method (y). $S_{y \cdot x}$ is determined by least square linear regression for each of three data
levels: low, normal, and high. The ± $2S_{y \cdot x}$ distance is plotted upwards and downwards
at the midpoint of each of the subgroups, parallel to the y axis, from the line for the
whole range of data. These points are then connected by dotted lines.

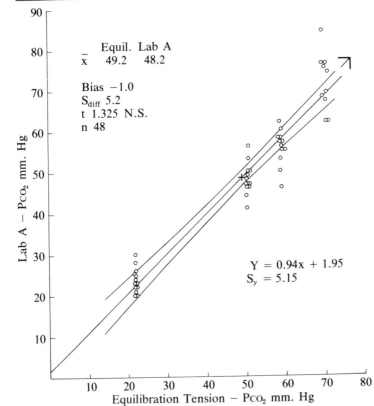

Figure 6-7
Confidence interval (CI) of line as a whole [4]. Data for Pco_2 by electrode (y) versus known equilibration Pco_2 (x) using four calibrated gases. Regression line by least squares. Confidence interval is enclosed by slightly divergent lines on either side of regression line. This situation can be visualized by imagining the line pivoting around the midpoint within the CI envelope, and can be described as the uncertainty of the true best line due to the smallness of sample size. For calculation details see Natrella [2], Chapter 5, pp. 15–17.

sample size are required for more precise estimates. Those who require frequent calculation of linear regressions will find that Natrella's format is easily programmed [2]. She also provides excellent algorithms for calculation of the confidence interval of the line as a whole, and of confidence intervals for future average values of y.*

Figures 6-6 and 6-7 compare straight-line graphs of various linear regression

*The confidence interval (CI) for future *average* values of y answers the following question: For repeated values of the same x_i, what is the CI of the mean value of y_c? The CI of a mean is determined from the standard error as $S_{y \cdot x}/\sqrt{n}$ data pairs. Roughly ± 2 such intervals is the CI of

methods which we have found useful. Of particular interest, Figure 6-7 provides a display of regression data replicated at a few points rather than the typical scattergram.

Pitfalls of Linear Regression

Linear regression may lead to serious misinterpretation of the data if you don't keep your wits about you.

Like the arithmetic mean, the regression equation without an estimate of the variance (such as $S_{y \cdot x}$) gives information which is useful but incomplete. The range of the data is critical. Values which have a narrow numerical range, such as serum sodium, yield regression equations with wide confidence bands; this causes uncertainty as to the true location of the line. A general rule is that a range in which the highest value is less than three times the lowest tends to be misleading. An alternative approach requires the ratio s population/s method to be greater than 10. Furthermore, the artificial introduction of a few high or low values when most values cluster in the center will not solve the problem. When values are concentrated in the center, paired t-test statistics (see Chapter 15) are the proper choice. Much like children on a seesaw, extreme values have a disproportionately large effect on the position of the line. One possible procedure is to omit from analysis values beyond three standard deviations from the mean. The effect of extremes is quite similar to that described in the section on the correlation coefficient.

Similarly, because the extremes of the line are generally less certain than the middle regions, be skeptical of predictions of y values much beyond actual observed data.

In addition, the least squares method has a particular deficiency worth mentioning. It presumes that x is known precisely and that all variability of measurement is confined to y. This assumption is usually appropriate when x represents such precisely measured factors as temperature and mass, but it is usually not true when we compare most of our laboratory methods with each other. When the imprecision in the measurement of x is attributed entirely to the y values, the effect is to reduce the slope. The group averages method does not suffer from this defect, but it does require much more complex programming for unbiased estimates of m and b [1].

Various forms of weighted regression techniques are designed to compensate for the effects of range, frequency, and the imprecision of x on least squares. Textbooks on regression mathematics should be consulted by those interested.

---

the future average values of y. Another useful calculation is the CI of the line as a whole, as illustrated in Figure 6-7, indicating indecision as to the exact position of the true line. This type of analysis is particularly useful for calibration curves, as exemplified for HiCN in Table 6-1 and Figure 6-5. By plotting the data for a number of monthly calibrations one finds a confidence interval envelope. If a subsequent calibration line failed to fit close to this envelope one could suspect difficulty with the standards or the photometer.

However, the best way of safeguarding against misinterpretation is to understand the limitations of the data.

Linearizing Functions

Because the mathematics of linear equations are simple to use in hand calculations and small programmable computers, nonlinear functions are often converted to linear functions. Large lists of such transformations are available.

Two nonlinear functions frequently found in the clinical laboratory are exponential curves and power curves. These are transformed to linear expressions by conversion to logarithms. A brief review of logs may be useful for those who have forgotten how to use them. The word logarithm stems, quite appropriately, from the Greek words for logic (reason) and for arithmetic. A logarithm is basically an exponent. A logarithm to the base 10 (abbreviated $\log_{10}$ or simply log) refers to the exponent or power to which 10 must be raised to yield a certain number. For example, the $\log_{10}$ of 100 is 2.000 because $10^2 = 100$. Similarly, the log of $1,000 = 3.000$.

Because logs are really exponents, adding them together is the same as multiplying the two original numbers. Likewise, when logs are subtracted from each other it is the same as dividing one original number by the other. And when two logs are multiplied it is the same as raising the number 10 to the power of the product.

The term *antilog* refers to the original number whose log is a certain value. Thus the antilog of 3 is 1,000, because 1,000 is the number whose log is 3.

Sometimes you may find references to *natural* logarithms. These are logarithms based on e, the number $2.7183+$. They refer to exponents of e and may be symbolized as $\log_e$ or ln. The number e appears as a limiting value in differential calculus and holds great fascination for mathematicians.

An exponential curve, when plotted on semi-log paper, yields a straight line. Such a curve can be linearized by a logarithmic transformation:

$$y = (a)(10^{kx})$$

$$\log y = kx + \log a$$

We then solve by converting y values to logarithms and by using the logs of y and the x values in the transformed equation.

$$\log y = k\ x + \log a$$
$$\downarrow \quad \downarrow\downarrow \quad \downarrow$$
$$y = m\ x + b$$

In this arrangement, the slope is k and the y-intercept is $\log a$. Next, take the antilog a. Substitute k and antilog a into the equation $y = (a)(10^{kx})$, the original form of the equation, from which y_c's are calculated and $S_{y \cdot x}$ then derived.

Thus, if k is .95, antilog a is .12, and a given (x,y) pair is (2,9), then

$$y_c = .12 \ (10^{.95 \times 2}) = .12 \ (10^{1.9}) = .12 \ (79.43) = 9.53$$

Then, $y - y_c = -.53$. By setting up a table similar to Table 6-2, $S_{y \cdot x}$ can be calculated as shown.

Data which become linear on log-log paper follow a power curve and are linearized by the following transformation:

$$y = (a)(n^x)$$
$$\log y = n \ (\log x) + \log a$$
$$\downarrow \quad \downarrow \quad \downarrow \qquad \downarrow$$
$$y = m \quad x \quad + b$$

Convert x and y values to their logs. Slope $= n$ and y-intercept $= \log a$. Substitute the value of n and the antilog of a in the original form of the equation, $y = (a)(n^x)$, and proceed with the calculation of y_c's and $S_{y \cdot x}$.

One type of common laboratory data which follow an exponential curve is study of quantitative immunoglobulins by immunodiffusion. Many coagulation factor assays follow power curves.

The Correlation Coefficient (r)

This statistic is also known as Pearson's product moment. It permits us to judge how well two independent (bivariant) groups of measurements or observations tend to agree on a scale extending from -1 to $+1$. When r $= 1$, agreement is perfect; when r $= 0$, data are random with respect to each other; and when r $= -1$, agreement is perfectly inverse. Intermediate values denote mixtures of agreement and randomness.

It should be noted that the r value has no dimension. Practically anything can be correlated with anything. The values correlated can be as disparate as hair length growth per week versus Dow-Jones averages. A correlation coefficient, by itself, does not imply cause and effect.

A formula that is easily programmed and suitable for use with the tabulation made for linear regression (Table 6-2) is

$$r = \frac{n\Sigma xy - (\Sigma x)(\Sigma y)}{\sqrt{[n\Sigma x^2 - (\Sigma x)^2][n\Sigma y^2 - (\Sigma y)^2]}}$$

From the data in Table 6-2,

$$r = \frac{5,337.9 - 4,637.6}{\sqrt{(5,371.8 - 4,651.2)(5,309.2 - 4,624)}} = \frac{700.3}{702.67} = .9966$$

Frequently r values are given with a p value; i.e., r = +.7, p < .05. For the curious, this p value can be obtained from a *t*-test for r (is r really different from 0?):

$$t_r = \frac{r}{\sqrt{\dfrac{1 - r^2}{n - 2}}}, \quad df = n - 2 \ (x,y) \text{ pairs}$$

A useful property of r allows insight into the components of variance in the underlying linear regression. The square of r estimates the proportion of variability of y due to the variability in x (that is, x values in Table 6-2 vary from 3.1 to 11.0 with y tending to correlate). The remaining variance is a function of $S_{y \cdot x}$, the variance attributable to accidental, random, or unexplained deviations of y_c from the observed y values.

The mathematical expression justifying this property of y can be derived from the equation for r and from the linear regression equations as:

$$S_{y \cdot x} = s \text{ population } (1 - r^2)^{1/2}$$

if you are a good mathematician. Even if you are not, with a little college algebra and by converting the standard deviations to variances, you can see that

$$\frac{(S_{y \cdot x})^2}{(s_{pop})^2} = 1 - r^2$$

Thus, it is clear that the proportion of the whole population variance caused by method imprecision (randomness) can be dissected by this simple ANOVA from the variance due to the range of patient values selected for correlation.

The pitfalls of r are similar to the pitfalls of linear regression. A correlation coefficient of +.9 between methods may seem very good indeed, but remember, r = +.9 implies that almost 20 percent of the variance is due to intermethod randomness. Beware of the salesman who comes only with r's! In our laboratory a correlation coefficient of less than 0.995 between concentrations of standards and spectrometer absorbance for many analytes is rejected as a faulty calibration curve by our computer.

The correlation coefficient is also subject to the effects of range, outlying values having excessive influence and tending to improve the apparent r. Considering the example in Table 6-6, note how, without any change in the most clinically relevant region, the addition of an extreme upper and lower value improves the correlation coefficient between two methods for sodium.

In strict usage, correlation coefficients are not suitable for functionally related data such as those obtained from comparison of sodium or WBC by two methods. Such data ought to agree closely. However, r is correctly used to correlate independent variables which have only a statistical relationship (such as hair growth and Dow Jones averages). Knowing what the data are and what

Table 6-6
Effect of Range of Values on r in Comparing Methods A and B for Serum Sodium

Test No.	Method A	Method B	Method A	Method B
1	—	—	105	108
2	124	126	124	126
3	126	120	126	120
4	130	135	130	135
5	132	130	132	130
6	138	135	138	135
7	140	145	140	145
8	141	135	141	135
9	143	148	143	148
10	—	—	164	160
$\bar{x}$ =	134.25	134.25	134.3	134.2
	r = .85		r = .95	

they mean clinically will provide the means for avoiding errors of interpretation.

References

1. Bartlett, M. S. Fitting a straight line when both variables are subject to error. *Biometrics* 5:207–212, 1949.
2. Natrella, M. G. Characterizing Linear Relationships between Two Variables in Experimental Statistics. In M. G. Natrella, *Experimental Statistics* (National Bureau of Standards Handbook 91, Chapter 5). Washington: U.S. Government Printing Office, 1963, reprinted 1976.
3. Westgard, J. O., and Hunt, M. R. Use and interpretation of common statistical tests in method-comparison studies. *Clin. Chem.* 19:49–57, 1973.
4. Weisbrot, I. M., Kambli, V. B., and Gorton, W. L. An evaluation of clinical laboratory performance of pH-blood gas analyses using whole blood tonometer specimens. *Am. J. Clin. Pathol.* 61:923–935, 1974.

7 Sampling

Choice of a proper sample for study is one of the most critical decisions in statistics. If the sample is adequate any errors in statistical manipulations can be corrected later, but if the sample is inadequate no amount of statistical expertise can prevent the drawing of improper conclusions. Most medical misinformation is based on lack of care in sample selection.

We will illustrate this aspect of statistics by posing the question, What is the normal range for blood glucose?

Accurate Definition

This apparently simple question has many facets which must be decided *before* we embark on a large program of mass screening for diabetes and hypoglycemia. Starting from the laboratory angle, what method shall we use? We have previous knowledge that plasma glucose is higher than whole blood glucose; we also know that Folin-Wu methods yield consistently higher values and glucose oxidase methods consistently lower values than does the Somogyi-Nelson method. We must therefore choose both sample and method in advance; if we wish to derive independent estimates for these variables we must collect the proper information and subgroup the data appropriately. Suppose we decide to use a ferricyanide method and a plasma sample; we have eliminated several variables in advance and can handle the data as a whole, as far as the analytic technique is concerned.

Our next question could be, When should we draw the sample? We know that blood glucose rises after a meal and then falls, also that it is higher in the afternoon than in the morning. We must define these variables and collect data accordingly. We might collect only fasting morning samples, which would yield only fasting normal values; or we might indicate on our data cards the time of day and the number of hours after a meal. If our series were large enough we could break down the values into groups, such as two hours after breakfast, or one hour after lunch, and derive normal ranges for each. This sort of statistical analysis is simple for a computer although extremely tedious if done manually.

Another question relates to preceding diet. Subjects who have been starved may respond as if they were diabetic and, contrarily, subjects who eat too much candy are prone to hypoglycemia. We must therefore inquire as to previous diet. We might choose to omit any individual whose history suggested a peculiar diet immediately preceding the study, or we might segregate the values from these individuals and analyze them separately.

Having coped with these obstacles we must approach some even more difficult questions concerning the definition of *normal*. For some blood constituents there are different normal levels for males and females and for different age groups. We must certainly collect age and sex on the data cards and attempt to produce normal ranges for each subgroup. The size of the subgroups, such as 0 to 19 years, 20 to 60, and over 60 (or some other units), can be decided after the experiment by setting up contrasting grouping to observe whether a real difference exists. We know that blood glucose ranges are unequivocally higher in older persons, but now we encounter a philosophic question of serious import: Is this increase normal and unrelated to the health of individuals, or is it due to the inclusion of mildly diabetic individuals who will develop associated illnesses? Students of the subject are divided on this score, but in our experiment we must start with a definite plan, such as establishing ranges for each sex and age-related peer group.

Our next definition is that for the normal range. Shall we include 80 percent, 90 percent, or some other percentage of all individuals? Shall we first eliminate obvious "sick" values? If so, what criteria should be selected? Most often we set arbitrary cutoff limits to exclude outlying values, then define normal as the mean $\pm 2s$; this causes 4.55 percent of persons to be considered abnormal, about half being above and half below the acceptable range. Arbitrary as this system may be, it does give us well-defined guidelines.

Accurate Identification

Particularly in experiments of this kind in which many samples are processed, the problem of maintaining accurate specimen identification is important. We need not belabor the difficulties that arise when the specimen is not the one for which the data has been accumulated.

Sampling Techniques

In the example used so far we assume that the persons whose blood is drawn for glucose determinations are a random sample of the population, so that estimates of the ranges obtained could be accepted as representative of the population. This assumption may be wrong. For instance, we might be attracting known diabetics anxious for a free checkup. Usually, however, we can discount this error by follow-up studies, careful questioning, and so on, so that no serious bias is introduced. There are many other types of experiments, however, in which bias can be avoided only by advanced planning, using one of the techniques to be described.

Paired Samples

If we wish to study a single variable we may do this by carefully pairing our individual samples so that members of each pair will be identical except for the variable to be tested. In laboratory practice this is usually simple. We wish to compare the results of two methods for testing plasma glucose. We perform both methods on each sample and compare the results, preferably using the same technologist and certainly assuring ourselves that sample deterioration has not occurred.

For most therapeutic experiments it is not possible to use a single subject for different trials, and if it were possible we must recognize that the subject has been changed by the passage of time and by the effect of the first trial. We can cope with this difficulty by using paired subjects for trial, one-half of them being treated in sequence A then B; the other half, B then A. This eliminates the effect of the two variables—passage of time and sequence of trials. If we do pair subjects by preselection we must avoid the introduction of bias by the experimenter. If the sicker member of the pair always receives the treatment and the healthier one is the control, we are automatically discounting the possible therapeutic merits of the treatment. If pairing is to be done the selection for each therapy must be carried out in a systematic fashion, as described in the later section on Latin squares, to assure that each variable is equally weighted.

Randomization

When we randomize a series we make use of a tool which is of much wider application than pairing. We assure ourselves that choice of treatment, for instance, is selected entirely at random with no choice by the experimenter or the patient. When all the studies are properly tabulated and completed we can then analyze the data for the effect of each variable with considerable confidence that the results were not preordained by the experimental design itself. There are many ways in which randomization can be performed, but the one most generally utilized at present is by using tables of random numbers (see Appendix Table 1). These numbers have been scientifically selected to be

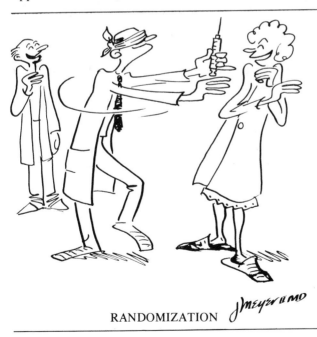

RANDOMIZATION   Meyer II MD

perfectly random. To use them in an experiment for dividing a group into two subgroups (e.g., treatment and no treatment) we can start anywhere in the table. Take the first number in the left upper corner (for instance) and assign it to the first patient who appears. The next patient receives the second number, going either horizontally or vertically. We continue in this fashion until all the individuals are assigned. One must skip numbers already used. If one group is larger than the other, we can cope with this statistically. Patients with odd random numbers will be used as one subgroup, and those with even numbers as the other. There are an infinite number of ways of using random number tables, and the example shows only a single method.

Why is assigning random numbers more reliable than merely assigning sequential numbers (1, 2, 3, 4, . . .) as the patients appear? Because under some circumstances there may be actual selection at work in the sequence of patients. In one famous example patients who were admitted to treatment were alternated by day of admission; those who appeared the first night received treatment A, the second night treatment B, the third night treatment A, and so on. When this became obvious to the medical community, each referring physician admitted his patients on the appropriate night to receive the treatment he preferred; the two series were therefore selected in advance and were not random at all.

"Blind" Techniques

"Blind" techniques make use of variables which are not made known at the time of the experiment. The "double-blind" method commonly used in therapeutic trials is designed so that neither the subject nor the therapist knows which regime is being utilized for each patient. This is not always easy and is sometimes impossible; some medications, for example, have a characteristic taste, odor, or side effect which is not found in the control or placebo. The difficulty of assuring proper controls should not persuade one to ignore certain basic precautions.

PATIENT SUGGESTIBILITY. All patients are to some degree suggestible as regards both subjective and objective findings. About 40 percent in any series have some effects from placebos which have no known physiologic effects. Certain diseases and certain symptoms are particularly associated with a high degree of suggestibility. In one study in which I participated a group of chronic sufferers from rheumatoid arthritis were chosen for study because their names had been in the clinic files for years and they were receiving no treatment. At the time of the first visit they were carefully examined, a comprehensive history was taken, and blood was withdrawn for sedimentation rate measurement. At the time of the next visit a week later each one volunteered that he felt much better! This fine therapeutic response to no specific therapy is a clear warning of the need for careful controls.

OBSERVER SUGGESTIBILITY. All observers are to some degree suggestible. Consciously or otherwise, they may wish an experiment to succeed or fail. The less the observer knows about the expected result the more dispassionate and objective he can be.

DUPLICATE OBSERVATIONS. Repetition of observations is useful only if the observer does not know the first result. Duplication of known observations, one after the other, is futile. This will be discussed at greater length in Chapter 12, Duplicate Measurements.

Sample Size

It is self-evident that the larger the sample, the more representative of the whole population it will be—*if it is well-chosen.* A good little sample is much better than a bad big sample! It is also self-evident that the larger the sample, the more work is involved in carrying out each aspect of the study and the more expensive it will be. We therefore ask, What is the smallest sample size we would choose to answer our questions effectively? Unfortunately there is no single answer for all questions. Two examples will clarify this.

1. How can it be determined if a new drug causes thrombosis? (This has been a critical area in evaluation of contraceptive pills.) If untreated women have an incidence of 1 case of thrombosis per 20,000 per year [2] and if the medication produces 9 cases per 20,000 per year, it is apparent that many thousands of cases must be studied to state reliably that there is such an increased incidence.

2. In dealing with acute childhood leukemia a medication is administered and a permanent cure is achieved. Can this medication be recommended on the basis of one favorable experience? Of course; if there had never previously been a cure of leukemia, then one genuine cure would be very encouraging!

Thus an experiment may be useful with one case or may require thousands. The latter situation occurs particularly when idiosyncrasies to drugs are involved. Fortunately for most other patient purposes, where statistics are applicable, series of 40 or 50 comparisons are adequate.

When dealing with alternatives, the relevant formula is

$$s = \sqrt{\frac{pq}{n}}$$

where n = total number of cases

p = percentage of positive findings expressed as a decimal

q = percentage of negative findings expressed as a decimal ($q = 1 - p$)

Suppose we consider that there is an equal chance that a treatment will or will not have an effect ($p = 0.5, q = 0.5$). We test this hypothesis by treating 50 patients. s (expressed as a decimal) will be

$$\sqrt{\frac{0.5 \times 0.5}{50}}$$

or 0.071. Our 95 percent confidence limits for 50 trials are 25 ± (2 × .071 × 50), or 25 ± 7.1, or 17.9 to 32.1. If less than 17 or more than 32 patients improve we reject the hypothesis at the 5 percent probability level, so the treatment has exerted an effect, either harmful or helpful!

Another example more closely related to laboratory testing is in the evaluation of blood smears. Suppose several persons do differential leukocyte counts on the same smear. How closely will their counts agree, assuming each picks an area of satisfactory cell mixing?

Our relevant formula again is

$$s = \sqrt{\frac{pq}{n}}$$

Suppose the lymphocytes are actually 40 percent of the cells and each person counts 100 cells.

$$s = \sqrt{\frac{.40 \times .60}{100}} = \sqrt{\frac{0.24}{100}} = \sqrt{.0024} = .049$$

$s = 4.9$ percent; $2s = 9.8$ percent, so the limits are $\bar{x} \pm 2s$, and 95 percent of counts will fall between 30 percent and 50 percent. We could narrow these limits by counting more cells. For a 500-cell differential the $2s$ value would be

$$\frac{9.8}{\sqrt{5}}$$

or 4.4, so 95 percent of counts would be between 35.6 percent and 44.4 percent.

Unfortunately our original premise for any experiment may be wrong, as happens quite frequently. We have no way of predicting this, so we set up a trial in an arbitrary fashion. The size of the trial series is predicated on the difficulties. If we were trying the effects of a dangerous surgical procedure we would limit the size as much as possible; if we were comparing automated laboratory tests each costing a few cents we could start with a large series.

Our conclusion when we compare the two series, test and control, is either:

1. We do not have convincing evidence of any difference between the two series, or
2. We have demonstrated a difference between the two series at a probability level of .05, or .01, or some other figure.

When we care carrying out comparisons in which numerical values rather than yes or no answers are to be obtained we rely on t tests to determine the significance of differences. Because we usually don't know the size of the differences we anticipate, we may have to guess what size series is needed. On the other hand, we can preselect a difference that we consider significant and work out a sample size exactly.

Suppose we analyze blood glucose by method A, whose s was 5 mg., or by method B, whose s was 3 mg., and we would consider a difference in mean values of 4 mg. as the maximum acceptable. We take a t value of 2.0 as probably being appropriate at the .05 probability level. Our formula is

$$t = \frac{\text{acceptable difference } \sqrt{n}}{s \sqrt{2}}$$

where n = number of differences
$\quad s$ = standard deviation of the method with the larger s.

Substituting,

$$2.0 = \frac{4\sqrt{n}}{5\sqrt{2}}; \quad n = 12.5$$

When we check our t table for 13 df at the 5 percent probability level we find the critical value to be 2.160. If we use this value instead of 2.0 for t in the formula, n becomes 14.6, so we need 15 pairs to assure ourselves of the .05 probability that the means are really different. If we reversed our question we might ask whether 50 pairs, yielding 50 df, would be adequate to detect a difference of 4 mg. in the mean values for methods A and B. We substitute:

$$t = \frac{4\sqrt{50}}{5\sqrt{2}} = 4.0$$

For 50 df our t table value is 2.008 (5% level) and 2.678 (1% level), both much less than 4.0, so we could be very confident in the results of 50 paired analyses.

Multiple Variables

There are many ways of handling multiple variables to be studied in a single sample. Obviously the original data must clearly specify each variable so that the series can be broken down into contrasting groups. If a well-randomized experiment has been done, each variable can be studied by analysis of variance (Chapter 5). Special arrangements are also possible, as the following suggests.

Latin Squares

Latin squares are another approach to analysis of multiple variables. A prearranged diagram is used to plan the experiment so that the maximum data can be extracted from a small series of studies. The key to this is "balance," requiring some data in each cell for each combination of variables, thus forcing the selection of balanced samples. This technique is best explained by the following example taken from work we performed some time ago [1].

We were concerned with discrepancies between the results of prothrombin tests performed at different times by different technologists, and we wondered whether an instrumental technique would cut down obvious discrepancies when it was substituted for a manual method. We decided to perform comparisons both on normal specimens and on those with a prolonged prothrombin time. Finally, because we knew that prothrombin times become longer when specimens age, we wanted to be sure that specimen deterioration did not affect our experiment.

We first confirmed the fact that there was no bias between the Fibrometer and tilt-tube methods on 40 clinical samples, using a statistical scheme previously described. We then set up the following plan:

1. Four experienced medical technologists were chosen to perform the experiments; their initials were O., L., W., and N.
2. Four Latin squares were designed (Table 7-1). Note that the order of performance for each person and each specimen was different for each day. It was this feature which permitted each factor to be analyzed separately.
3. Each technologist received a form for each day of the experiment. He was called in the proper sequence by the Chief Technologist, performed the four analyses, recorded the values on the form, and submitted the data to the Chief Technologist. The values entered by each analyst were unknown to the others. The data were filed and not analyzed until the entire experiment was completed.
4. The Chief Technologist picked four specimens for each of four days, two in the normal range and two in the high range, from the routine prothrombin time tests. Every specimen was ample to provide a sample for each participant. All analyses of each specimen were completed within 20 minutes of one another. Every specimen received a 2-digit code number, the first digit indicating an arbitrary specimen number and the second digit indicating the day of the experiment.
5. On the first day, the Fibrometer was used; on the second day, the tilt-tube; on the third day, the Fibrometer; and on the fourth day, the tilt-tube.

Note that this technique permitted each analyst to examine one specimen first, one second, and so on, for each series of tests; that each specimen was analyzed first once, second once, and so on, in each series; and that by

Table 7-1
Latin Square Design
Order of Performance

	Technologist			
Specimen*	O.	L.	W.	N.
11	1	2	3	4
21	2	3	4	1
31	3	4	1	2
41	4	1	2	3
12	2	3	4	1
22	3	4	1	2
32	4	1	2	3
42	1	2	3	4
13	3	4	1	2
23	4	1	2	3
33	1	2	3	4
43	2	3	4	1
14	4	1	2	3
24	1	2	3	4
34	2	3	4	1
44	3	4	1	2

*Last digit in specimen number indicates day the specimen was tested.
Source: Barnett and Pinto [1] (© 1966 by Williams & Wilkins Co., Baltimore, Md.).

rearranging the data we could analyze each factor separately, as indicated in Tables 7-2, 7-3, and 7-4.

In Table 7-2 the data are rearranged for maximal utility. The horizontal columns are arranged in order of performance. The last column gives the arithmetic mean for each specimen and the arithmetic mean of the greatest ranges for each specimen. The arithmetic mean of performance by each of the 4 technologists for each group of specimens is listed in Table 7-3.

Table 7-4 lists the pooled estimate of standard deviation between technologists and was calculated as follows: In each category of four specimens (normal values obtained with the Fibrometer, normal values obtained with the tilt-tube, and so on) the arithmetic mean for each specimen was determined. The difference (d) between each individual value and the mean for that specimen was then calculated and squared. For the four specimens there were 16 such squared values (d^2) and all were added together. The sum of the 16 values was divided by 12 (because there were four specimens, each with 3 degrees of freedom). The pooled standard deviation was then determined by taking the square root of the sums of the squares divided by 12 according to the formula

Table 7-2
Latin Square Design
Results in Order of Performance

Category	Specimen No.	Order of Performance				Greatest Range
		1st	2nd	3rd	4th	
		sec.				*sec.*
1. Normal values, Fi-brometer	11	11.9	11.8	12.4	12.4	0.6
	21	12.4	12.3	12.4	12.3	0.1
	13	13.9	13.9	13.9	13.9	0.0
	23	13.4	13.4	13.4	13.5	0.1
Mean of 4 specimens		12.90	12.85	13.02	13.02	0.20
2. Normal values, tilt-tube	12	13	11	15	12	4
	22	12	13	12	14	2
	14	14	13	13	14	1
	24	14	16	15	14	2
Mean of 4 specimens		13.25	13.25	13.75	13.50	2.25
3. High values, Fibrom-eter	31	27.9	29.4	29.9	29.9	2.0
	41	19.8	20.4	20.5	19.9	0.7
	33	25.9	26.9	27.9	27.4	2.0
	43	30.4	32.3	32.3	33.9	3.5
Mean of 4 specimens		26.00	27.25	27.65	27.77	2.05
4. High values, tilt-tube	32	26	25	26	24	2
	42	28	27	26	26	2
	34	38	38	38	39	1
	44	33	35	36	37	4
Mean of 4 specimens		31.25	31.25	31.50	31.50	2.25

Source: Barnett and Pinto [1] (© 1966 by Williams & Wilkins Co., Baltimore, Md.).

$$s = \sqrt{\frac{\Sigma d^2}{n}}$$

where n = degrees of freedom.

Upon inspection of Table 7-2 in a horizontal direction, no evidence of deterioration of specimens during the time of the experiment is found in categories 1, 2, or 4. There is some suggestion of such deterioration in Category 3, High values, Fibrometer. This experiment was repeated subsequently and the following mean values were obtained for 4 specimens examined by 4 technologists: specimen examined first, 30.88; second, 31.25; third, 31.10; and fourth, 30.25.

From these values, which show no deterioration, and from use of the Wil-

Table 7-3
Latin Square Design
Performance by Technologists
Mean of 4 Values for Each

Technologist	Level of Prothrombin Values	Fibrometer (*sec.*)	Tilt-Tube (*sec.*)
O.	Normal	12.90	12.75
L.	Normal	12.87	14.75
W.	Normal	13.00	13.00
N.	Normal	13.00	13.25
Range among technologists		0.13	2.00
O.	High	27.00	31.50
L.	High	27.22	32.00
W.	High	27.52	30.75
N.	High	26.92	31.25
Range among technologists		0.60	1.25

Source: Modified from Barnett and Pinto [1] (© 1966 by Williams & Wilkins Co., Baltimore, Md.).

Table 7-4
Latin Square Design
Pooled Estimate of *s* among Technologists*

Level	Fibrometer	Tilt-Tube
Normal	0.165	1.127
High	0.974	1.118

*Four specimens in each category.
Source: Barnett and Pinto [1] (© 1966 by Williams & Wilkins Co., Baltimore, Md.).

coxon rank-sum* test for the combined samples, we concluded that there was no deterioration of samples in Category 3.

The comparative precision of the two methods is as follows: In the normal range, the Fibrometer is capable of much greater reproducibility between technologists, as determined by the much smaller mean range between technologists (0.13 second) than that obtained with the tilt-tube (2.00 seconds), and by the much smaller pooled estimate of *s* between technologists (0.165 second) than that obtained with the tilt-tube (1.127 seconds).

On the other hand, there is no significant difference between the precision of the two methods in the abnormal, high range (range of the mean between

*A nonparametric statistic (see pp. 9 and 227).

technologists, 0.60 versus 1.25, pooled estimate of s between technologists, 0.974 versus 1.118).

From inspection of tubes containing the coagulum formed during the two methods, it seems that the explanation of the differing results at various levels of activity is as follows. In the normal range a good, solid clot is formed instantaneously at the end point; differing readings in manual methods are almost entirely due to differing criteria of clotting and technologist reaction time. The instrument all but eliminates these differences. In the high range the coagulum is tenuous and forms gradually so that the end point is truly indeterminate by any method, except within rather broad limits.

Data obtained in this fashion can be subjected to a variety of comparisons with considerable assurance that each variable is properly controlled.

Besides Latin squares there are many other arrangements for the systematic handling of several variables, but these are outside the scope of this volume.

References

1. Barnett, R. N., and Pinto, C. L. Reproducibility of prothrombin time determinations between technologists. *Am. J. Clin. Pathol.* 46:148–151, 1966.
2. Vessey, M. P., and Doll, R. Investigation of relation between use of oral contraceptives and thromboembolic disease. *Br. Med. J.* 2:199–205, 1968.

8 Bayesian Statistics

The Bayesian theorem is concerned with the probabilities of mutually exclusive events. Because this theorem has enjoyed a recent vogue, and because the problem dealt with is common both in the study of patients and in the medical laboratory, we will discuss it briefly. A typical problem to which it can be applied is illustrated in Table 8-1.

Table 8-1
Frequency of a Particular Symptom in Two Diseases in 500 Patients

| | Symptom X | | |
Disease	Present	Absent	Total
A	60	40	100
B	140	260	400
	200	300	500

Source: From D. Mainland, Statistical ward rounds—5 (*Clin. Pharmacol. Ther.* 8:738–748, 1967).

The probability that when symptom X is present, disease A is also present is

$$p(A|X) = \frac{p(X|A)p(A)}{p(X)}$$

The vertical bar indicates "when present," i.e., $p(A|X)$ means probability that A is present when X is present.

Substituting values from Table 8-1,

$$p(A|X) = \frac{0.6 \times 0.2}{0.4} = 0.3$$

because X is present in 60/100 of A; A is present in 100/500 of all patients; and X is present in 200/500 of all patients.

This is called *frequentist* Bayesian statistics and has certain obvious merits in deciding the usefulness of laboratory procedures.

A different use of the Bayesian formula is called *subjectivist*. The formula becomes

$$p(H|D) = \frac{p(D|H)p(H)}{p(D)}$$

where H stands for the hypothesis and D for data. $p(H)$ is then the prior probability of a hypothesis expressed mathematically. This formula gives an apparent scientific-mathematical aura of respectability to an "educated guess." Its value is debatable and we will not discuss it further. (For further discussion see D. Mainland, Statistical ward rounds: 5. *Clin. Pharmacol. Ther.* 8:738–748, 1967).

II Application of Statistics in the Clinical Laboratory

9 Normal Values

In Chapter 7, Sampling, we considered the establishment of normal values for a large population and discussed some effects of methodology, time of drawing the sample, preceding diet, sex, age, presence of sick persons in the group, definition of the normal range, and sample size. In this chapter some of these and related matters are discussed in more detail.

The term "normal values" has been severely criticized. Substitutes proposed to modify the term "values" (and also ranges, limits, or intervals) have included "customary," "reference," "referent," "critical," "functional," "representative," "standardized," "predictive," "expected," "conventional," "optimal," and "innocuous," with the further modifier "clinical" frequently added. Nevertheless, because "normal values" has been used conventionally for many years and because the term is familiar to most clinical personnel, we will continue to use it—without claiming any merits other than customary usage.

Developing Normal Ranges

When I first directed a clinical laboratory and physicians would ask, "What is your normal value for constituent X?" I would reply, haughtily, "The same as everyone else's, of course!" I have since learned that this answer was approximately 100 percent wrong. Unfortunately, many laboratories still report normal ranges culled from the literature, oblivious to all the differences in all the variables between their values and those of other laboratories. Frequently these ranges are not altered when new methods are adopted, even though these may be very different. *It is essential that every laboratory develop its own normal values for every test commonly used.* For unusual tests ranges must still be taken from the literature, but with great care to identify them as such and to use the same method as the one published.

Effect of Methods

The precision of the method used has a measurable effect on the apparent normal range. If we assume that there are two variables in the measured population range, namely, the method of measurement and the population, we can visualize the ANOVA formula:

$$s^2 \text{ (measured)} = s^2 \text{ (method)} + s^2 \text{ (population)}$$

We can use this as a tool for determining the contribution of each factor. Suppose that for plasma glucose the measured s of the population is 11 mg., $\bar{x}$ is

106 mg., and the known s of the method is 5 mg. Substituting in the formula,

$121 = 25 + s^2$ population.

then s^2 (population) = 96 and

s (population) = 9.80.

The true population range, expressed as $\bar{x}$ (106) ± 2s (19.60) is then 86.4 to 125.6 mg. Our measured range was $\bar{x}$ (106) ± 2s (22.0) or 84 to 128 mg. The imprecision of the method widened our measured spread from 39.2 mg. to 44 mg., or by a factor of 44/39.2 = 1.12, or by 12 percent. Suppose we improved our technique so that s (method) became 2 mg. instead of 5 mg. Assuming the true population range were still 86.4 to 125.6, what would our new measured range be? We again substitute in the formula

$$s^2 \text{ (measured)} = s^2 \text{ (method)} + s^2 \text{ (population)}$$

$$= 4 + 96 = 100$$

and s (measured) = $\sqrt{100}$ = 10

Our measured range of $\bar{x}$ (106) ± 2s (20) becomes 86 to 126. This is a 40 mg. spread, as compared to our original measured spread of 44 mg.; it is thus 40/44 or 91 percent of the original spread. Under these conditions a great effort to improve the method has not yielded correspondingly great returns in identifying abnormal values.

For a contrasting example let us consider serum calcium.

s (measured) = .5 mg./100 ml., $\bar{x}$ = 9.2, s (method) = .4.

Substituting,

$0.5^2 = 0.4^2 + s^2$ (population),

then s^2 (population) = 0.3.

The apparent range as measured is $\bar{x}$ (9.2) ± 2s (1.0) or 8.2 to 10.2. But the true range was $\bar{x}$ (9.2) ± 2s (0.6) or 8.6 to 9.8. The apparent spread/true spread relationship of 2.0/1.2 is 167 percent of the true spread because our method is crude. If we could improve our method to an s of 0.2, we could narrow the measured range very significantly, assuming the population range remains as calculated.

Then s^2 (measured) = $0.2^2 + 0.3^2$

$= .04 + .09 = .13$

and s (measured) = .36

Then the range of $\bar{x}$ (9.2) $\pm$ 2 s (.72) becomes 8.5 to 9.9 mg., or 1.4 mg., compared to the previous 2.0 and the true 1.2 mg. This has almost eliminated the contribution of methodology to increasing the measured range. Therefore a substantial effort to improve calcium methodology would be warranted if we wished to narrow the normal range and identify abnormal values more effectively.

This approach to the problem is useful for pinpointing the tests whose precision needs improvement. Because in practice we cannot dissociate the method from the population, we must consider the normal range as including both variables.

When we compare normal ranges in different laboratories, the bias of the method becomes crucial. Even when two laboratories perform a test by allegedly following the same method in every detail, including a common source of standards and reagents and the same instrumentation, it is unusual for them to achieve identical results. The results today are becoming more uniform because of external quality control programs and proficiency surveys, so bias within the same method is becoming less important; nevertheless we cannot currently rely on this to avoid the necessity for finding local normal ranges.

When a laboratory changes methods, new normals probably should be established, even if there appears to be no change in the results as judged by a comparative study of the old and new methods. (See Chapter 15.) This will obviate unexpected problems at the low and high limits of the normal range.

Selection of Population

It is axiomatic in statistics that a sample should be as representative as possible of the population from which it is derived. If possible, then, we should attempt to establish normal ranges for age, sex, and perhaps racial groups, controlled as to time of day, inpatient or outpatient status, and any other variables we can identify. If we succeed in this elaborate endeavor, how do we decide which subjects represent an ill population as regards the substance under test? We can identify them on either statistical or collateral grounds, neither of which is entirely reliable.

On statistical grounds we might start by excluding all values beyond $\pm$ 3s or even $\pm$ 2s of the mean and by assuming the remainder to be the normal population; or we could handle the data in a similar manner through the use of percentiles. This system may exclude persons who do not have any evidence of illness related to the abnormal value and who may never develop such an illness. Contrariwise, if we examine persons with these "abnormal" levels and find no disease, we have no assurance that they will not develop an illness related to the abnormal value.

Alternatively, we might select only persons who were job applicants, or blood donors, or candidates for elective minor surgery, and who had no discernible illness, and confine our sample to these persons. Would they be

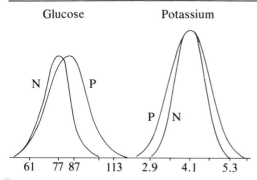

Figure 9-1
Distribution of values from 50 student nurses (N) and 500 consecutive patients (P) by Hoffman's method. Note that for potassium the means are identical but the patient range is wider; for glucose the patient mean is 10 mg. higher, the range also wider. Glucose in mg./100 ml. Potassium in mEq./L. (From R. N. Barnett, Interpretation of laboratory data. *Israel J. Med. Sci.* 2:519–524, 1966.)

reasonably comparable to persons who were generally ill and confined to bed for illnesses not related to the constituent under analysis? The effect on the normal range of using the two systems just described is portrayed in Figure 9-1.

Amador and Hsi [1] have considered the subject in detail, comparing normal ranges derived from normal ambulatory persons with those calculated by six "indirect" (patient population) methods, and finding them substantially different for most serum constituents. Unfortunately this does not solve the following basic questions: Should we evaluate values for hospital patients in the same context as those for normal ambulatory persons? Would our diagnoses and treatments be better, or might we indeed cause harm? These are medical, logical, and philosophic rather than statistical questions, and they cannot be answered by statistical methods.

It has been proposed [2] that we accept the narrow range of truly healthy young people as ideal and attempt to influence everyone's levels into these ranges; but at this moment I believe such an approach is premature and that we do best by using as the appropriate sample peer groups from which we statistically eliminate outliers.

The size of the sample needed was discussed in Chapter 7. If we work with carefully chosen groups a sample size of 40 is usually adequate, but in using a system based on consecutive hospital patients, Hoffman [4] recommends 500 as the standard series. This allows for effective separation of the "sick" values from the "healthy" ones.

One rarely discussed aspect of normal ranges is the need for periodically reviewing them. Certainly when methods are changed, particularly if new chemical principles are used, it is necessary to recalculate the ranges. Even if methods remain apparently the same it is possible for new personnel, standards, or reagents to alter the results. Less obvious, however, is the actual change in the population over the years. We accept the fact that in each generation Americans grow taller and heavier, so that our normal values for size have been altering constantly. However, there are only a few studies of clinical laboratory values sufficiently reliable to compare defined groups at different times. One of these [6], apparently based on good evidence, indicates that 24-hour thyroidal radioiodine uptake fell from 28.6 percent in 1959 to 15.4 percent in 1967–68 in the same population of euthyroid patients. This is a very significant change.

Calculating Normal Values

The simplest method to calculate normal values, using a selected, apparently normal population, is as follows:

1. Calculate $\bar{x}$ and s by the formulas

$$\bar{x} = \frac{\Sigma \text{ of values}}{n} \qquad s = \sqrt{\frac{\Sigma(x - \bar{x})^2}{n - 1}}$$

2. From this data set a range of $\bar{x} - 3s$ to $\bar{x} + 3s$.
3. Eliminate from the original data any values which are outside these limits.
4. Recalculate $\bar{x}$ and s from the remaining values.
5. The accepted normal range is then $\bar{x} \pm 2s$, using the values in step 4. This includes 95.45 percent of values and excludes the highest 2.27 percent and the lowest 2.27 percent, if the values are distributed in a normal distribution curve.

Use of Normal Probability Paper

If unselected values from a hospital population are utilized to calculate normal ranges, it is necessary to separate the normal from the "sick" components. This can be done by plotting values on graph paper and superimposing a normal distribution curve (Figure 9-2), or by plotting on normal probability paper, which transforms the normal curve into a straight line. In either case we first group the data in classes in ascending order as in Table 9-1.

We may now plot this data as in Figure 9-2. On regular graph paper we plot glucose levels on the abscissa and the number of values at each level on the ordinate. (Note that we put the number of values opposite the level of the midpoint of the class—e.g., for 85 to 89 we use 87, and for 90 to 94 we use 92.) We then draw an actual curve fitting all the points. It is evident that there are two modes. We assume that the left-hand peak represents the normal population. By eye we then draw a normal distribution curve symmetrically, using the left side as a model; the dotted line is the projection of the right side of this

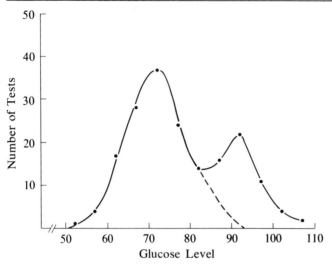

Figure 9-2
Calculating normal range on ordinary graph paper from patient values listed in Table 9-1. All values plotted by classes. Upper curve includes all data. Dotted line is projection of normal distribution curve plotted by eye to match opposite side of curve. $\bar{x} = 72$, range 56 to 88 ($\bar{x} \pm 2s$) for normal part of distribution curve.

Table 9-1
Calculating Normal Range
Blood Glucose (mg./100 ml.), Data Arranged by Classes in Ascending Order

Level (mg./100 ml.)	Number of Samples	Cumulative Number	Cumulative Percent
45–49	0	0	0
50–54	1	1	0.6
55–59	4	5	2.8
60–64	17	22	12.2
65–69	28	50	27.8
70–74	37	87	48.3
75–79	24	111	61.7
80–84	14	125	69.4
85–89	16	141	78.3
90–94	22	163	90.6
95–99	11	174	96.7
100–104	4	178	98.9
105–109	2	180	100.0

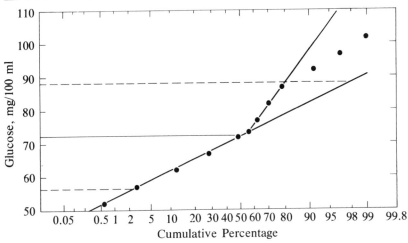

Figure 9-3
Calculating normal range on normal probability paper from patient values listed in Table 9-1 using cumulative percentage column. The lower plotted line is drawn through the lower 6 points and projected. The horizontal lines are drawn from the intersection of the plotted line with 2.5%, 50%, and 97.5% lines. The plotted line for points 7, 8, and 9 in ascending order indicates a second population. The uppermost 3 points are not connected because they represent too few determinations. The three horizontal lines intersect the glucose values at 56, 72, and 88 mg., indicating $\bar{x} = 72$ (solid line), range = 56 to 88 ($\bar{x} \pm 2s$) indicated by broken lines.

normal curve. From observation of the points of inflection we find the lower limit at 56, the mean at 72, and the upper limit at 88.

Alternatively we use probability paper (Figure 9-3). We list the glucose levels on the ordinate; the abscissa is already marked off as cumulative percentage. Using the class midpoints we plot the cumulative percentages from the table. We then draw a straight line representing the normal distribution, using the lower values. Note that at 73 mg. the observed values depart from the straight line, and for illustration we have drawn a line through the next 3 points, indicating another population. The upper 3 points we ignore because they represent so few individuals. Using the normal distribution line we now connect to the ordinate line from the 2.5 mark, giving a lower limit of 56, the 50 mark giving a mean of 72, and the 97.5 mark giving an upper limit of 88. (These are the lines connected to the ordinate.) These values are about the same as those we derived from the previous graph; either method is ordinarily adequate.

Another method which avoids any assumptions about the normal distribution of values is the percentile method of Herrera [3]. She recommends use of the

Table 9-2
Calculating Normal Range by Percentiles
Blood Glucose (mg./100 ml.), Single Values Listed in Ascending Order

Rank	Value	Rank	Value	Rank	Value	Rank	Value
(1)	69	(6)	73	(11)	80	(16)	85
(2)	70	(7)	76	(12)	80	(17)	87
(3)	70	(8)	76	(13)	83	(18)	89
(4)	72	(9)	78	(14)	83	(19)	90
(5)	72	(10)	79	(15)	84		

tenth and ninetieth percentiles rather than 2.5 percent and 97.5 percent. The method is as follows:

1. List all values in ascending order, the lowest being No. 1 (rank 1).
2. Take 10 percent of $n + 1$, n being the total number of values. This is the rank number of the tenth percentile. For example, if there were 49 values, $n + 1$ = 50, 10 percent of 50 is 5, so the fifth value in order would represent the tenth percentile.
3. The ninetieth percentile is found in the same way, with the *highest* number given rank No. 1. In the example given it would be the fifth number from the highest.

The sample of 19 glucose values in milligrams per 100 ml. is given in Table 9-2 merely to illustrate the technique, *not* to recommend such a small sample. Take 10 percent of $19 + 1 = 2$. The tenth percentile then is No. 2, 70 mg.; the ninetieth is No. 18, 89 mg.

See Table 9-3 for estimating the limits of population excluded for different sample sizes, as done by Herrera [3]. This table is used as follows: For example, take sample size 79. The tenth percentile value found in a series of this size represents, almost every time, actual population values between percentiles 4.47 and 17.42. In only 5 percent will this tenth percentile value be outside of these limits; in only 2.5 percent will it fall below the 4.47 percentile and in only 2.5 percent will it exceed the 17.42 percentile.

Log Normals

Periodically there is a wave of enthusiasm for the notion that for some or many body constituents the population distribution is log normal rather than as indicated by a normal distribution curve. This is particularly true for substances like bilirubin, whose normal value is near 0, so that a normal curve gives some negative results. Inasmuch as excessively low values for such substances are not accurately determined nor of any clinical significance, the establishment of

Table 9-3
Use of Percentiles in Calculating Normal Range*

Sample Size	Limits of Percentage Excluded	
	Lower	Upper
19	1.30	26.00
29	2.19	22.78
39	2.87	20.89
49	3.39	19.61
59	3.83	18.69
69	4.17	17.97
79	4.47	17.42
89	4.73	16.94
99	4.95	16.56
109	5.15	16.22
119	5.31	15.93
129	5.47	15.67
139	5.62	15.46
149	5.75	15.27
159	5.86	15.07
169	5.98	14.91
179	6.07	14.76
189	6.16	14.62
199	6.25	14.50
209	6.29	14.38

*Illustrates 0.975 probability limits for different sample sizes.
Source: From L. Herrera, The precision of percentiles in establishing normal limits in medicine (*J. Lab. Clin. Med.* 52:34–42, 1958).

a "correct" lower limit is of no use even if the distribution is truly log normal. Actually the standard deviation is such a robust tool that it is not much affected by moderate changes from the usual bell-shaped curve.

If it is desired to determine log normal distribution the procedure is simple. A table is made up in which classes are separated, as just described. The log of each class midpoint is then taken and the log classes are plotted on either ordinary graph paper or probability paper. The mean and 95 percent limits are determined as if the log values were actual values. They are then converted back to actual values to yield the "correct" range. In a log normal distribution the mean is nearer one end than the other of the range (Figure 9-4). It can be seen that as long as the upper limits are the same, the interpretation of single patient values as being normal or not will be identical, regardless of the shape of the curve. A value of 0.85 is within normal limits and one of 1.0 is excessive, either way.

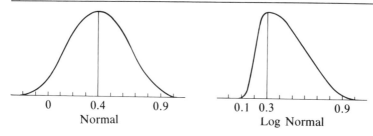

Figure 9-4
Identical data on bilirubin values in mg./100 ml. are plotted as a normal distribution in left-hand curve and as log normal distribution in right-hand curve. Note that the normal curve goes below zero, which is obviously impossible. $\bar{x} + 3s$ upper limit is 0.9 mg./100 ml. and is the same by either method.

Gram-Charlier Analysis

Martin, Gudjinowicz, and Fanger [5] have performed exhaustive studies on normal values and have concluded on clinical, mathematical, and statistical grounds that use of Gram-Charlier series is a more satisfactory technique than either the Gaussian or percentile models described above in separating out the abnormal component from a mixed population. Curves which are asymmetric (skewed) can be analyzed by this technique. The analysis requires a large computer and extensive programming; therefore there is no reason to describe the statistical manipulations or the mathematical theory here. In essence the process analyzes a large number of results (about 300 to 500), determines whether there is only one population or several, and then calculates the range for each population. A point is found that best separates the normal from the abnormal range, and this is called the minimum error sum point.

Because of the frailties of any mathematical model, it is essential to validate the minimum error sum point based on actual clinical studies. A number of patient charts are selected in which the test values fall close to the critical level chosen; generally about 10 percent of the total number of values, half above and half below the breakpoint, are chosen. For example, let's take the actual values for SGOT,* the Gram-Charlier analysis and the illness probability and error sum results shown in Figures 9-5 and 9-6. The minimum error sum appears to be at about 30 units on Figure 9-6. We therefore check 35 charts whose SGOT value in the study ranged from 26 through 34.

The charts are then reviewed using all the available information *except* the test result, which should be concealed. If the point was chosen properly there should be mostly normal patients (for the analyte) on the normal side of the minimum error point and mostly abnormal patients on the abnormal side. A simulated example of these values appears in Table 9-4.

*Serum glutamic oxaloacetic transaminase.

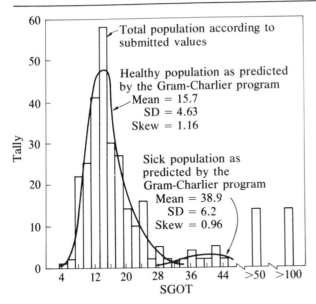

Figure 9-5
Analysis of 297 admission SGOT values by Gram-Charlier program. Note the two populations; most of those in the sick population have alcoholic liver disease.

Note the good but not perfect fit in which normal individuals are more numerous at low SGOT levels and sick individuals are more numerous at higher levels. Given the difficulties in chart evaluation and the analytic variability of enzyme methods, these figures are strong evidence to support the minimum error point of 30.

We can also use Figure 9-6 and the chart analysis in another productive fashion. Suppose that we are interested in using the SGOT analysis for excluding myocardial infarction. We wish to be very certain that we do not miss any cases, and we are willing to accept a few "false positives." We could then set our cutoff point at, for example, 24 units rather than 30. This would make the probability of detecting the disease by this test about 97 percent rather than 72 percent, although it would increase the error sum from 3 to 5. Alternatively, if we were screening an alcoholic population for definite liver damage and didn't want to include any dubious cases, we could set the cutoff point at 40 units.

Cole [2] has approached the problem in a similar but more tedious fashion. He reviewed numerous charts from persons whose blood urea nitrogen (BUN) value was known, and he established the critical level using the type of data shown in Table 9-4 as his only statistical tool. When Martin took this original data and performed a Gram-Charlier analysis on 965 of the cases, he found essentially the same BUN level dividing normals from abnormals. This proved most encouraging in establishing the statistical model as a valid one. The

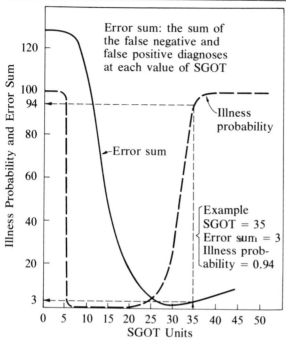

Figure 9-6
Further analysis of same 297 admission SGOT values portrays error sum and illness probability for individual SGOT values.

Table 9-4
Illustration of Test Results on Charts Chosen for Evaluation of Minimum Error Sum Point Following Inspection of Figures 9-5 and 9-6

| | | On Basis of Patient Evaluation: | |
Number of Patients	Test Result	Test Result Should Have Been Normal	Test Result Should Have Been Abnormal
6	26	6	0
9	28	6	3
7	30	4	3
8	32	3	5
5	34	1	4

College of American Pathologists is currently attempting to provide this type of analysis as a practical laboratory tool.

Portraying Normal Ranges

Because the normal range is usually used in medicine to help determine the state of health of individuals, it must be available for the decision-making process. The simplest scheme is the publication of a normal range on the laboratory report form itself. The physician then compares the patient value to the range and decides whether it is normal, low, or high. The interpretation of abnormal values is discussed in the Patient Care section (Chapter 18). Unfortunately, even the most sophisticated reports presently generated do not specify normal values for peer groups; this should be a real asset for computer-generated printouts, which can be programmed to provide the proper range for each group of patients. Printed ranges based on local data are a great advance compared to ranges taken from the literature or the physician's memory. One difficulty is the ease with which abnormal results may be overlooked because the medical attendant is so deluged with numbers; the present situation is deplorable [9] and will doubtless get worse as more and more tests are done for each patient.

Various methods of calling attention to abnormal results are in use. Some computers identify abnormal values with an asterisk. Attempts to use a different color printout have not proved practicable so far. One study group [9] put an opaque dot over each abnormal result, requiring the physician to pull it off to see the figure!

Another approach is the use of graphic readouts as presently generated by several widely used automated analytic devices. The normal range is indicated by a crosshatched band or other system, and the patient value appears as a line either within or without the normal range. This is an effective device for attention-getting. There are proposals [7] to have the computer print a graphic display in which deviations from the normal are portrayed visually rather than numerically.

The ideal situation, which can be achieved within a few years, will be a computer printout of all data that will indicate the peer group range for the laboratory and will call attention in some effective fashion to abnormal values.

References

1. Amador, E., and Hsi, B. P. Indirect methods for establishing the normal range. *Am. J. Clin. Pathol.* 52:538–546, 1969.
2. Files, J. B., Van Peenan, H. J., and Lindberg, D. A. B. Use of "normal" range in multiphasic testing. *J.A.M.A.* 205:94–98, 1968.
3. Herrera, L. The precision of percentiles in establishing normal limits in medicine. *J. Lab. Clin. Med.* 52:34–42, 1958.

4. Hoffman, R. G., and Waid, M. E. The "Average of Normals" method of quality control. *Am. J. Clin. Pathol.* 43:134–141, 1965.
5. Martin, H. F., Gudzinowicz, B. J., and Fanger, H. *Normal Values in Clinical Chemistry: A Guide to Statistical Analysis of Laboratory Data.* New York: Marcel Dekker, 1975.
6. Pittman, J. A., Dailey, G. E., III, and Beschi, R. J. Changing normal values for thyroidal radioiodine uptake. *New Engl. J. Med.* 280:1431–1434, 1969.
7. Rushmer, R. F. Accentuate the positive. *J.A.M.A.* 206:836–838, 1968.
8. Werner, M., and Cole, G. W. *Urea* (Clinical Chemistry Critique No. CC-106). Chicago: American Society of Clinical Pathologists, 1977.
9. Williamson, J. W., Alexander, M., and Miller, G. E. Continuing education and patient care research: Physician response to screening test results. *J.A.M.A.* 201:118–122, 1967.

10 Quality Control

Maintenance of a satisfactory level of performance has been a primary goal in clinical laboratories for many years. This control of quality has many facets. First, the individual ingredients of the test procedure must be as excellent as possible. These include supplies, reagents, instruments, and personnel. Second, the samples themselves—blood, urine, or whatever—must be handled carefully. Finally, the process itself must be carried out correctly and the results reported accurately and on the correct sample. A satisfactory quality control program must concern itself with each of these facets.

For many of the tests yielding quantitative results it is possible to study the output as an index of the reliability of the whole process. This concept, originally developed for industrial products by W. A. Shewart of the Bell Telephone Company, was first applied to the clinical laboratory by Levey and Jennings in 1950 [9] and later popularized by Copeland [4]. A number of systems exist for such an evaluation and are discussed here individually.

Stable Samples

In this category we include frozen pooled serum, lyophilized serum, and stable cell or particle suspensions. The material chosen is analyzed repeatedly at intervals. Following this, calculations are made to determine the mean, standard deviation, and confidence limits. Once this has been accomplished a sample is analyzed with each batch of tests; the analytic value should fall within the confidence limits chosen.

Types of Stable Material

The first material used was frozen pooled serum, and this is still frequently employed. It is prepared as follows: Each day after the analyses are completed the remaining clear, nonicteric serum free of hemolysis is poured into a large (2 or 3 liter) flask which is kept in the freezer at $-20°C$. When the desired amount—usually that expected to last for 3 to 9 months—has been accumulated, it is processed. It is thawed, thoroughly mixed, filtered through glass wool, aliquotted in stoppered containers of appropriate size, and refrozen. This type of specimen has the advantages of being cheap and easily produced, being of human origin, and requiring no dilution. The major disadvantage is that certain constituents are not stable, particularly high levels of enzymes and CO_2. These substances fall for some time, then level off at a low level and remain stable. In addition, calcium values which are stable for several months later fall slowly and erratically. The following constituents remain stable for 9 months or more: glucose, urea, phosphorus, cholesterol, total protein, albumin, globulin, chloride, sodium, potassium, bilirubin, creatinine, uric acid, and low levels of the following: amylase, transaminase, lactic dehydrogenase, and alkaline phosphatase.

Special pools may be prepared by freezing serum with special desirable properties. For example, high bilirubin pools can be prepared from serum from jaundiced patients; material from exchange transfusions of very icteric infants is especially useful. Protein-bound iodine (PBI) pools at various levels are made from serum already analyzed for PBI rather than from random specimens, in order to exclude those very high values often found after injection of organic iodides. Because precision and accuracy differ at different levels, it is often desirable to use two pools, one normal and one high for certain constituents. For some substances it will be found that s is constant at all the usual levels, or alternatively that CV is constant at all these levels. If this is true there is no necessity to use two pools. If there is no consistent relation one then makes the two pools, preferably at or near decision levels of medical significance.

Hemoglobin control material is readily prepared from hemolyzed whole blood and is stable if kept sterile. Unsterile hemoglobin solution deteriorates rapidly even when frozen. Our own technique follows: Two 500 ml. donor bottles containing freshly drawn human blood in A.C.D. (acid citrate dextrose solution) are emptied into large, sterile centrifuge bottles and spun down. The supernatant plasma is aspirated completely and a more or less equal volume of sterile distilled water is added to cause hemolysis. The bottles are shaken on a mechanical shaker for 30 minutes. They are then placed in a freezer at $-20°C$ for 24 hours, removed, thawed to room temperature, and filtered through a Millipore filter into a sterile flask. The hemoglobin concentration is tested and adjusted to about 10 gm./100 ml. by adding distilled water if necessary. A magnetic stirring bar is placed in the flask and the solution mixed for 30 minutes. Then, using a blood administration IV set with filter and a siphon mechanism, 1 ml. aliquots are aspirated into vacuum tubes and frozen. They remain stable for over a year.

All of the "homemade" preparations described above are potential sources of infectious hepatitis viruses. To diminish this hazard, each batch should be tested by the most current test for such viruses before being added to the large pool, and all batches giving a positive reaction should be eliminated. Commercial materials described below have already been tested and found free of demonstrable viruses.

Another stable product is lyophilized serum, widely available from many commercial sources. It is the only satisfactory source of high range enzyme material which does not remain stable in liquid serum. The values listed by the producer are used as guides to the general level but should not be accepted as gospel, because enzyme methods, even those using the same specified technique, are not identical. Enough material of the same lot should be purchased to last a number of months. There are a number of disadvantages to this material. First, it is frequently of animal origin and may give anomalous reactions in enzyme determinations. Second, it requires reconstitution with diluent, providing a source of error not present in frozen serum. Finally, it is moderately expensive. Properly used, particularly for small installations, this material is very satisfactory. There are a number of groups and state organizations all using the same batches of commercial material for quality control purposes. This has the advantage of providing a basis for comparison with the peer group, besides providing confidence limits for each participant.

Additionally, there are available particle suspensions of several types for use in cell counting. These include latex particles, pollen particles, and preserved cells. For erythrocyte counting these materials provide a reasonable facsimile of ordinary erythrocytes. Unfortunately, stable leukocyte suspensions are not available; simulated material such as preserved nucleated avian erythrocytes is not ideal because the erythrocyte hemolysis necessary to ordinary leukocyte counting cannot be carried out.

Statistical Manipulations

Using any form of stable material, the statistical handling of data is simple. In the usual design a single sample of material is analyzed once a day for 20 days. It is imperative that the material be thoroughly thawed if frozen, accurately diluted if necessary, and thoroughly mixed to assure uniformity. The once-a-day framework is chosen because this is the commonest usage in the clinical laboratory; that is, the physician orders a test, gives a treatment, and the next day checks the result of his treatment. If analyses are carried out more frequently, the variation among results will be smaller and will portray a spurious illusion of precision. In general, within-day variation is one-half that of day-to-day variation.

Having tabulated the 20 values, we calculate the mean and the standard deviation, using either of the two formulas described in Chapter 5. We then prepare a chart in which the mean is the center line, the upper line is $\bar{x} + 3s$, and the lower line $\bar{x} - 3s$. The examples given in Tables in 10-1 and 10-2 illustrate the technique.

Graph

Whichever system of calculation is used, the mean $= 102.1, s = 3.01, 3s = 9.03$, upper control limit $= 111.13$, lower control limit $= 93.07$. A graph prepared using these figures and plotting the points given in the examples is shown in Figure 10-1.

The choice of $\pm 3s$ limits gives us a confidence of 99.73 percent that any deviation outside these limits is not the result of chance alone and therefore indicates genuine breakdown in the procedure. If we were to choose $\pm 2s$ limits, which some analysts use, our confidence is only 95.45 percent and we would expect an out-of-control value about once in 22 days instead of once in 384 days. This means that if 22 materials are in the quality control program we can expect one out-of-control value almost daily. The result is either that excessive amounts of time are spent in checking chance variation or that the

Table 10-1
Quality Control of Glucose Pool (mg./100 ml.)
Values for 20 Days, 1 per Day
Method One

Specimen No.	Date	Value	Difference from $\bar{x}$	Difference^2
1	10/8	98	4.1	16.81
2	10/9	102	0.1	0.01
3	10/10	108	5.9	34.81
4	10/11	110	7.9	62.41
5	10/13	102	0.1	.01
6	10/14	100	2.1	4.41
7	10/15	102	0.1	.01
8	10/16	104	1.9	3.61
9	10/17	100	2.1	4.41
10	10/18	104	1.9	3.61
11	10/21	100	2.1	4.41
12	10/22	98	4.1	16.81
13	10/23	102	0.1	.01
14	10/24	102	0.1	.01
15	10/25	104	1.9	3.61
16	10/27	102	0.1	.01
17	10/28	102	0.1	.01
18	10/29	102	0.1	.01
19	10/30	98	4.1	16.81
20	10/31	102	0.1	.01
		$\Sigma = 2,042$		$\Sigma d^2 = 171.80$

$\bar{x} = 2,042/20 = 102.1$
Divide Σd^2 by $n - 1$ (19) = 9.042
Take square root = 3.007 = s

Note: Calculated by formula $s = \sqrt{\dfrac{\Sigma(x - \bar{x})^2}{n - 1}}$.

technical staff pays little or no attention to out-of-control values. I therefore recommend the 3s limits as being the most practical.

The occurrence of seven or more points in a row on the same side of the median line is highly unlikely to be the result of random variation. This is a clear-cut warning that some systematic error has entered the system.

Expanded Calculations: ANOVA

Amenta [1] illustrated an expansion of this type of quality control system which involves more analyses (two samples a day, distributed randomly in the run, for 25 days) and which permits the derivation of additional information. Using this

Table 10-2
Quality Control of Glucose Pool (mg./100 ml.)
Values for 20 Days, 1 per Day
Method Two

Specimen No.	Date	Value	Value^2
1	10/8	98	9,604
2	10/9	102	10,404
3	10/10	108	11,664
4	10/11	110	12,100
5	10/13	102	10,404
6	10/14	100	10,000
7	10/15	102	10,404
8	10/16	104	10,816
9	10/17	100	10,000
10	10/18	104	10,816
11	10/21	100	10,000
12	10/22	98	9,604
13	10/23	102	10,404
14	10/24	102	10,404
15	10/25	104	10,816
16	10/27	102	10,404
17	10/28	102	10,404
18	10/29	102	10,404
19	10/30	98	9,604
20	10/31	102	10,404

$$\Sigma x = 2{,}042 \qquad \Sigma x^2 = 208{,}660$$

$$\bar{x} = \frac{\Sigma}{n} = \frac{2{,}042}{20} = 102.1 \qquad (\Sigma x)^2 = 4{,}169{,}764.0$$

$$\Sigma x^2 = 208{,}660.0$$

$$\frac{(\Sigma x)^2}{n} = 208{,}488.2$$

$$\text{difference}\left(\Sigma x^2 - \frac{(\Sigma x)^2}{n}\right) = 171.8$$

$$s^2 = \frac{\text{difference}}{n-1} = \frac{171.8}{19} = 9.042$$

$$s = \sqrt{9.042} = 3.007$$

Note: Calculated by formula $s = \sqrt{\dfrac{\Sigma x^2 - \dfrac{(\Sigma x)^2}{n}}{n-1}}$

mg/100 ml

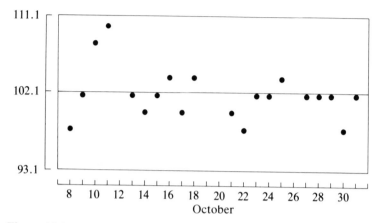

Figure 10-1
Quality control chart for glucose plotted from data in Table 10-1. $\bar{x} = 102.1$ mg.; $\bar{x} \pm 3s$ range is 93.1 to 111.1.

data and ANOVA, as described in Chapter 5, one can calculate the individual contributions to total variability that are contributed by place in the run, day-to-day changes, and residual method error. Control charts are made for overall limits, as in the conventional method, and also for day-to-day ranges. The advantage of being able to ascertain those components in greatest need of improvement is evident, but I am not confident that it is generally necessary. The following abbreviated example illustrates the ANOVA technique in detail (Table 10-3).

1. Calculate correction factor (CF) for mean of 20 values; this is

$$\frac{(\Sigma x)^2 \text{ for } A + B}{20} = \frac{33,014.89}{20} = 1,650.7445$$

2. Total sum of squares of deviations (x_t) (total variation) from overall mean is
$\Sigma x_t^2 = \Sigma x^2$ sample $A^2 + \Sigma x^2$ sample $B^2 - CF = 833.9100 + 817.5600 - 1,650.7445 = .7255$.

3. To divide this total into its components, first take day-to-day variation (x_D)

$$\Sigma x_D^2 = \frac{\Sigma x^2 \text{ for } A + B}{2} - CF$$

$$= \frac{3,302.21}{2} - 1,650.7445$$

$$= 1,651.1050 - 1,650.7445$$

$$= .3605$$

Table 10-3
Quality Control of Calcium Pool (mg./100 ml.) Using ANOVA
2 Determinations* Daily for 10 Days. Raw Data with Calculations of
Means and Sums of Squares

Day	Sample A	Sample B	$\Sigma(A + B)$	$\Sigma(A + B)^2$
1	9.0	9.4	18.4	338.56
2	8.9	8.7	17.6	309.76
3	9.3	9.2	18.5	342.25
4	9.1	9.0	18.1	327.61
5	9.1	9.0	18.1	327.61
6	9.3	8.9	18.2	331.24
7	9.2	8.9	18.1	327.61
8	8.9	9.2	18.1	327.61
9	9.5	9.1	18.6	345.96
10	9.0	9.0	18.0	324.00
Σx	= 91.3	90.4	181.7 Σx^2 = 3,302.21	
$\Sigma x/n$	= $\bar{x}$ = 9.13	9.04	9.085	
$(\Sigma x)^2$	= 8,335.690	8,172.160	33,014.8900	
$(\Sigma x)^2/n$	= 833.569	817.216	1,650.7445	
$\Sigma(x^2)$	= 833.910	817.560	3,302.2100	

*Carried out by atomic absorption.

4. The next component is position in the run (x_p) (see Table 10-3):

$$\Sigma x_p^2 = \frac{(\Sigma x)^2 A + (\Sigma x)^2 B}{10} - CF$$

$$= \frac{8,335.69 + 8,172.16}{10} - 1,650.7445$$

$$= \frac{16,507.85}{10} - 1,650.7445$$

$$= 1,650.7850 - 1,650.7445$$

$$= .0405$$

5. Finally, the residual error is what remains. $(x_r$ = remainder):

$$\Sigma x_r^2 = \Sigma x_t^2 - \Sigma x_D^2 - \Sigma x_p^2$$

$$= .7255 - .3605 - .0405$$

$$= .3245$$

Entering the F table for days (9 df numerator and 9 df denominator), the significant value at the 5 percent level is 3.18, so 1.111 is not significant; for

Table 10-4
Quality Control Using ANOVA
Final Calculations

Category	Σx^2	df	s^2	F
Total (t)	.7255	19	.03818	—
Between days (D)	.3605	9	.04005	1.111
Position in run (p)	.0405	1	.04050	1.123
Remainder (r)	.3245	9	.03606	—

samples (1 df numerator, 9 df denominator) the significant value is 5.12, so 1.123 is not significant (Table 10-4). We conclude that random variability, day-to-day variability, and between-sample variability are all about equally important. We now calculate our quality control graphs as follows to show both within-day variations (range) and day-to-day fluctuations.

First we need $\bar{x}$ and $2s$ limits. The mean for all 20 values is 9.085. s for the averages of 10 pairs is

$$\sqrt{\frac{s^2_D}{2}} = \sqrt{\frac{.04005}{2}} = \sqrt{.020025} = .14151$$

Our limits are to be set at $\bar{x} \pm 2s$ or 9.085 $\pm$ .283, namely 8.802 to 9.368. The standard deviation of the range between each two values is $\sqrt{2s_r^2}$ or $\sqrt{2} \times .03605$ or $\sqrt{.07210}$ or .2685. Inasmuch as the two values should be equal, the range should be 0 $\pm$ $2s$ or $-.537$ to $+.537$. Finally, the standard deviation for each measurement is $\sqrt{s^2 t}$ or $\sqrt{.03818}$ or .1954.

The graphs appear as shown in Figure 10-2. On inspection it appears that for the 10 days charted, both the averages and the ranges have remained within control.

If the range exceeds the acceptable limits there are random errors creeping in. If the average is out of control a systematic error is presumed to be operative.

Average of Normals

Hoffman's system [6] for calculating normal values for unselected population groups (Chapter 9) can also be used for quality control. The normal range is first calculated as described by finding the normal distribution of normal values and from this calculating the mean and standard deviation. Normal range in this system is considered $\bar{x} \pm 2s$. The standard error of the average for groups of normal values is derived as SE $= \dfrac{s}{\sqrt{n}}$, in which n is the usual number of normal values in a group. One then calculates confidence limits for groups of 16 values (Hoffman, 1967—a revision [personal correspondence] of his 1965 arti-

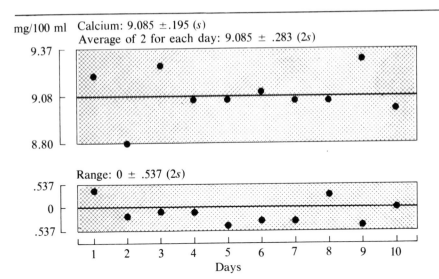

Figure 10-2
Quality control chart for calcium using ANOVA plotted from data in Tables 10-3 and 10-4. Upper lines indicate $\bar{x} \pm 2s$ limits for average of the two analyses in each run. Lower lines indicate range between first and second samples calculated as $\bar{x} \pm 2s$, in which $\bar{x}$ should be zero. The standard deviation on top of the chart is that for single analyses.

cle), using $\pm$ 2 SE limits. Choice of 2 SE limits rather than 3 SE limits makes the method more sensitive and assures more frequent out-of-control values. The analyst may grow to accept these outliers as being meaningless because they are so frequent; actually, if there are two in a row, or more than one a month, further investigation is necessary.

Having defined the limits we then take all the normal values (as already defined) each day and find the mean. The more values in the run the more effective the average becomes in defining the true range, as indicated in Table 10-5.

Table 10-5
Average of Normals
Probability of Detecting Error in Method with 95% Probability

Shift in s	Corresponding Shift in $\bar{x}$	10 Tests	16 Tests
0.50	0.39s	.27	.41
1.00	0.72s	.74	.90
1.50	0.99s	.95	.99

Source: Hoffman and Waid [7].

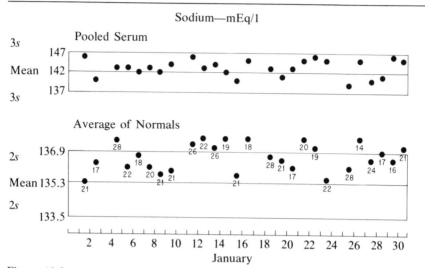

Figure 10-3

One month of values for sodium (mEq./L.). The numbers on the dots in the average of normals area refer to the number of normal values that were averaged that day. Pooled serum results are all in control though they appear somewhat higher than expected. Average of normal values are almost all high and frequently out of control. Actual calculations indicate that the pooled values for the month average 1.153 higher than expected and the average of normal values 1.163 higher. This excellent agreement is typical of a change in instrument performance which had actually occurred. The sensitivity of the average of normal values system is clearly shown.

This table expresses the likelihood of detecting a systematic bias which has entered the method. The magnitude of the shift in the mean is expressed in terms of the absolute value of s. For example, if $\bar{x}$ were 100 and s were 5, an actual upward shift of $1s$ or 5 units would produce an observed shift of only $.72s$ or 3.6 units, because some values previously excluded as being too high would now be included. There would be a .74 probability of detecting this shift through the appearance of an outlier in the graph if 10 patient samples were studied, and a .90 probability if 16 samples were included.

If there are less than 10 normal values in a run it may be wise to bring together values from two days to get a meaningful number.

There has been considerable controversy concerning the merits of this system, most of the criticisms being directed at its insensitivity. We do use it in collaboration with the pooled serum, as illustrated in Figure 10-3. One of its greatest merits is that it reflects the whole analytic process from the time the tourniquet is placed on the arm until the final result is reported. This gives a truer picture than the pooled serum, which is independent of patients. For example, we have detected the following changes in procedure only by the average of normal values method:

1. Change in procedure with tourniquets: tourniquets formerly left in place until sample drawn (correct); changed to removal of tourniquet followed promptly by aspiration of sample (incorrect)
2. Change in vacuum sample tubes to wrong kind
3. Progressive accumulation of dirt in AutoAnalyzer tubing—did not affect pooled serum, probably because of viscosity factors

Use of Patient Constants

For certain hematologic values Dorsey [5] recommends the use of patients' normal constants. This was necessary when no stable cell suspensions or similar material was available, and it still has merit. The presumption is that cell constants for a group of normal persons should fall within a narrow range which can be used for quality control limits. Details are as follows:

Blood from at least 11 normal adults is required for each run. *Normal* is defined as meeting these specifications: erythrocyte count of 4,000,000 or more, or hematocrit of 36 percent or more; red cells normal on smear; mean corpuscular hemoglobin (MCH) between 26 and 32 inclusive, or mean corpuscular hemoglobin concentration (MCHC) between 32 and 36 inclusive. Hemoglobin must be determined. Under these conditions mean values of the 11 or more samples should have an MCH between 29 and 30, or an MCHC between 32 and 33; additionally the $\bar{x} \pm 2s$ range should approximate normal values. A quality control chart can be prepared using these limits.

Each run containing enough data is calculated for $\bar{x}$ and s; if either appears out of control, appropriate measures are instituted.

This system, as the two preceding ones, measures changes in mean values as well as in precision. Because two variables go into each calculated figure, there are more out-of-control values than one would ordinarily expect. For example, let us accept a normal hemoglobin as 15.4, s 0.17; RBC 5,000,000, s 170,000, MCH 30.8. If the hemoglobin is high by $2s$ (value 15.74) and the RBC low by $2s$ (value 4.66), the MCH becomes 33.77, which is out of control, although actual measurements of both constituents were in control. This is not a problem if errors are random, but the system is excessively sensitive to small consistent errors in opposite directions. Also the normal ranges used may be unrealistically narrow. Nevertheless this general plan is valuable.

Details of Quality Control in Hematology

IRWIN M. WEISBROT

Single-channel hemoglobinometers and cell counters pose few quality control problems. They may be monitored with stable hemoglobin pools and fixed cell suspensions that have shelf lives comparable to the pools used in chemistry. Statistics, as already described for use in chemistry, are suitable. In our laboratory we usually find that our own mean and standard deviation differ

Table 10-6
Determining Precision from Duplicate Measurements (S_{Dup})
Leukocyte Counts, 10 Specimens

Specimen No.	Pipette A	Pipette B	Difference	Difference^2
1	7,970	7,400	570	324,900
2	9,470	9,230	240	57,600
3	7,410	7,230	180	32,400
4	14,820	15,410	590	348,100
5	3,610	4,690	1,080	1,166,400
6	4,590	6,280	1,690	2,856,100
7	4,490	3,700	790	624,100
8	9,980	10,870	890	792,100
9	14,890	14,260	630	396,900
10	5,240	5,540	300	90,000

$$s = \sqrt{\frac{\Sigma d^2}{2n}}$$

$\Sigma d^2 = 6,688,600$

Divide by 20 $= 334,430$

$s = \sqrt{334,430} = 578.3$

somewhat from those of the manufacturer's label assay. It is best to establish your own mean and standard deviation for the standard Levey-Jennings plot. Of course, if your own mean and standard deviation are extremely different from the putative value it is necessary to investigate—clean apertures; check thresholds, vacuums, rates of flow; try new vials and lots; and don't hesitate to do chamber counts on the fixed suspensions and on some patient samples if a large discrepancy is being investigated. Evaporation from the control vials can occur abruptly or gradually, poor mixing can ruin a vial, and freezing is disastrous. Barring these difficulties the Levey-Jennings plot will give adequate information concerning the instrument.

But no quality control system is complete without some tests based on patient samples. We find the standard deviation of duplicates useful (see Table 10-6). Analyze five specimens at clinically significant levels, store them under appropriate conditions for a few hours or overnight depending on the stability of the constituent, and repeat the analyses. A CV_{dup} can be calculated from the s_{dup} using the mean of all the values as $\bar{x}$. The CV_{dup} of the patient specimens will undoubtedly be larger than the CV of replicate determinations done on stable pools. The same series of duplicate analyses can serve as a check on calibration drift as well as precision. By doing a paired t test between the first and second series of determinations the statistical significance of any bias can be determined. Even if the bias is not statistically significant but you note that day after day it is in the same direction (always lower than the day before or always higher than the day before) the instrument should be investigated for drift.

When a question of accuracy arises, it is necessary to do chamber counts and to consult your results on proficiency surveys. We have already discussed chamber counts and their errors in the section on Poisson distribution. Despite the relative imprecision, particularly if only one chamber is counted, chamber counting is the reference method because it depends on basic physical constants, i.e., volume and number of particles. When chamber counting is employed for this purpose, each element of the system must be carefully calibrated, including the pipettes and chambers. Four to eight individual chambers should be enumerated.

Multi-channel blood analyzers (such as the Coulter Model S) are often controlled by modified whole blood suspensions which are processed like routine patient specimens. These suspensions suffer from short-term and long-term instability, are critically sensitive to mixing and storing techniques, are expensive, and have too short a shelf life to allow a classical Levey-Jennings plot. Frequently, normal level and abnormal level suspensions do not intercalibrate. However, some States require the use of these suspensions in their inspection and accreditation protocols. We use suspensions from two different manufacturers. A single analysis is made with one brand before the morning run and with the second brand before the afternoon run. We plot these results as plus or minus deviations from the manufacturer's stated mean as the zero line. After a few days we may note that our values are clustering high or low with respect to the manufacturer's mean, but our mean level usually lies well within the label limits for the assay. Purchasing is arranged to overlap manufacturers and lots, so that one brand is at midlife when a new shipment of the second brand arrives. The standard deviation of these differences from the manufacturer's mean serves as an estimate of precision, without being affected by variations in the assay level of different lots.

During the run, each tenth or fifteenth patient specimen is repeated in order to permit a running check on precision and calibration by inspection. At the end of the day the calculations for standard deviations of duplicates and a paired t-test can be done on these running duplicates.

Manufacturers no longer consider their cell suspensions to be calibrators. Calibration should be performed using fresh patient specimens, with normal erythrocyte morphology, that are analyzed by well-controlled reference methods such as chamber counts or by use of an electronic digital cell counter with threshold controls.

Smoothed Averages

Of particular interest in the calibration control of multi-channel instruments has been the introduction of smoothed averages. The central limit theorem tells us that if we take the grand mean of the averages of many small unbiased samples from a very large population, this grand mean will approach the true population mean very closely. This tendency is true even if the means of a few of the small samples are by chance very far from the true mean. Also, the central limit theorem holds true independently of the shape of the distribution curve of the population.

Smoothing techniques attempt to modify the average of a small sample and combine it with a previously determined grand mean in such a fashion that the random departure of the small mean from the true population mean is minimized. If the process is successful the new grand mean will be unchanged. Only if the small sample has within it an inherent shift in calibration will the new grand mean be changed.

A variety of empirical techniques for weighting or modifying the small sample are possible. Among them are truncation (arbitrary discarding of the highest and lowest values), logarithmic transformation, reduction of the weight of the small sample mean through use of a decimal multiplier, or a combination of these techniques. Taking the average of normals is another commonly used smoothing technique. Recently the mode has been suggested as a tracking signal for calibration [10]. In the hematology lab the most successful of these smoothed averages has been the Bull-Elashoff moving average for control of the Coulter Model S [3, 8].

The process begins by establishing the true grand population mean on many hundred patient specimens. During this initial study, calibration is carefully controlled by reference methods. Fortunately, most laboratories will have grand means close to those published; that is, 90 femtoliters for MCV, 30 picograms for MCH, and 33.5% for MCHC.

The results of 20 consecutive patient samples form the basis of the small sample mean. In effect, the manipulating algorithm causes the values to be separated into minus and plus values above and below the grand mean, which is arbitrarily designated as $\overline{X}_B$. The square roots of these differences are taken, a step which will have the effect of compressing values very far away from the mean. The values for the square roots derived from the positive numbers and from the negative numbers are summed separately, each sum retaining its positive or negative sign. They are then added algebraically and the results divided by 20. This residue, which is usually quite small, is added algebraically to the grand mean, which now becomes the new grand mean ($\overline{X}_{Bi}$). This value is plotted on a chart above or below the previously established mean ($\overline{X}_B$). Unless disturbed by a biased run (such as a group of high MCV's from the chemotherapy clinic) it rapidly responds to shifts of calibration of 1 to 2 percent in two or three sample cycles.

Assuming that the population means for red cell indices are indeed constant, both calibration and accuracy are in a sense tied to a biological standard. In the Coulter system, changes in MCH may be due to the hemoglobinometer or the red cell counting system; changes in MCV may be due to dirty apertures or changes in the electronics; and MCHC is affected by all three determinations (MCHC $\cong \dfrac{Hb}{Hct} \cong \dfrac{Hb}{RBC \times MCV}$). Although the algorithm is designed to be run on-line with a computer, we have found the method quite suitable as an off-line quality control technique by using a small programmable computer with hand entry. Because time limitations preclude entering each group of 20 patient specimens, we select three runs of 20 during the day. Even this "truncated" truncation rapidly detects calibrational drift and has, on a number of occasions, detected diluents with incorrect osmolality. The latter is particularly important for the control of MCV because preserved cell suspensions do not respond as do actual blood specimens to changes in diluent osmolality.

Determination of Precision from Duplicate Measurements

For some perishable components of body fluids no stable control material is available, nor are there recognized body constants, yet we would like to have some means of quality control. Accuracy cannot be determined by duplicate measurements but must be calculated in some other fashion. (See Chapter 11, Standardization.) Precision can be calculated within a run by the performance of duplicate measurements, and from the precision the probable meaning of changes in values can be estimated from time to time.

Using leukocyte counts as an example, we start with a sample of anticoagulated whole blood, draw two separate pipettes, and count each as blind duplicates in the same run. We then list the values in two columns as shown in Table 10-6. We find the differences between members of each pair, ignoring signs; square the differences; add them; divide by 2n (n is the number of pairs), and take the square root to find the standard deviation. (We divide by 2n because each pair is an individual variable, and each member of the pair has its own variability.)

Having found the standard deviation of the differences between duplicates, we can use the data to plot a quality control chart for precision similar to the lower chart in the ANOVA expanded calculations example (Figure 10-2). The entry each day is the difference between two analyses made from the same sample. The chart limits are $0 \pm 2s$ (for the leukocyte example $-1,157$ to $+1,157$); out-of-control values indicate, with 95 percent confidence, the existence of outliers in the analytic system.

Determination of Precision from Mixed Samples

One problem with determination of precision from duplicate analyses is the tendency of duplicates to give closer values than would random samples. (See Chapter 12). A system for avoiding this, which has been evaluated by Barnett and Pinto [2] and which we currently employ, is as follows:

From a batch of specimens two are selected at random and designated A and B. Equal portions of each are removed and mixed together to form a new specimen C. Analyses are carried out on all specimens. We then tabulate the results as shown in Table 10-7.

Table 10-7
Determination of Precision from Mixed Samples

Substance	A	B	C	$\dfrac{A + B}{2}$	Difference*	Analyst
Glucose	102	110	108	106	+2.0	J. T.
Urea N	18	17	17	17.5	−0.5	J. T.
Uric acid	7.7	4.0	5.8	5.85	−0.05	L. R.
Creatinine	4.8	0.6	2.7	2.7	0	L. R.

*The difference is that between the value found for the mixed sample (C) and the theoretical value $\dfrac{A + B}{2}$.

To prepare quality control charts for precision determined by this method, we perform analyses on each of 40 days. The average difference ($\bar{d}$) for a single analysis is found by adding all the differences (omitting the signs) and dividing by 40. A control chart is then prepared in which the 50 percent line is $0.845\,\bar{d}$, the 95 percent line is $2.5\,\bar{d}$, and the 99.5 percent line is $3.5\,\bar{d}$ (Figure 10-4). The 95 percent line corresponds to the usual $2s$ and the 99.5 percent line to the usual $3s$ limits in other quality control systems. (These factors are chosen because the standard deviation of each analysis is 1.2533 times the average difference. The 50 percent line is 1.2533 times 0.674, the 95 percent line is 1.2533 times 1.96, and the 99.5 percent line is 1.2533 times 2.807. In turn the values 0.674, 1.96, and 2.807 are taken from cumulative normal distribution tables. For example, $\pm\,1.96s$ in the table excludes 2.5 percent of upper values and 2.5 percent of lower values.)

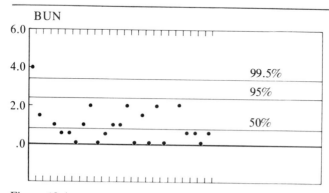

Figure 10-4
Distribution of differences in BUN analyses. Scale on ordinate in mg. Each point is the difference between the theoretical value calculated as an average of two samples and the actual value obtained by analyzing the mixed sample. The 50% line is $.845\,\bar{d}$; 95% line is $2.5\,\bar{d}$; 99.5% line is $3.5\,\bar{d}$. Note that only one result is outside 99.5% limits.

Each day that a mixed sample is prepared, a mark showing the d (difference) is placed on the chart as illustrated (Figure 10-4). If there are too many points above the 95 percent or 99.5 percent lines, appropriate investigations are carried out.

Comparison of Internal Quality Control Systems

We have now described five internal quality control systems. Three of them are capable of detecting systematic error; these are the stable samples, the average of normals, and the patient constants. The stable material probably has the widest application, but all of them have a useful place in the clinical laboratory. All detect changes toward higher or lower values, although none provides control of absolute accuracy. Most errors in clinical laboratories are systematic rather than random and reflect problems with reagents, standards, or techniques which tend to affect all rather than some samples. If such problems exist when limits for control charts are set, and if the problems continue, the system will not detect them. This is one reason why external quality control systems are so valuable (Chapter 14). For use in a single institution, however, the existence of a consistent bias may not be critical, but a changing bias may cause much harm. If charts indicate changing values, even if they are still within control, one should investigate promptly.

The systems which control only precision, those based on duplicates and those based on mixed samples, each have less to offer. In each of these the true values may be far wrong, but as long as the relative values are unchanged the system will not indicate the malfunction. Mixed samples have the merit of being unbiased, because no one knows the correct value for any of the three samples analyzed. We employ this system at least weekly and post the results for general inspection.

To what extent does conscious or unconscious bias affect results? If an analyst uses the same quality control material daily he soon learns the expected limits; potentially, this could lead him to falsify results if the specimen were out of control. In a study by Weinberg and Barnett [11] we found no evidence for this in our own laboratory. Nevertheless, I believe it does occur when extreme pressure of work exists or personnel policies are unfavorable. (One laboratory manager threatened employees with discharge if their quality control results were too poor—incompetence—or too good—dishonesty!) The mixed sample technique is effective in detecting overt sloppiness or dishonesty. Generally with modern automated and semiautomated methods there is little opportunity for "juggling" final results of individual tests.

Who should supervise and administer the quality control system? It should be someone in the routine laboratory itself, not in a separate department, because we are interested in actual performance as it relates to patient care. Although a specific "quality control" technologist may be employed to make sure that proper specimens are introduced, calculations carried out, and imme-

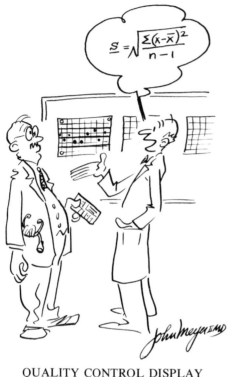

$$\underline{S} = \sqrt{\frac{\Sigma(x-\bar{x})^2}{n-1}}$$

QUALITY CONTROL DISPLAY

diate attention given to out-of-control values, this person should not perform the analyses under conditions differing from the routine used for patient analyses. Usually the chief technologist in the area supervises the program and delegates charting and calculations to others. With the small calculators and computers now available the calculations are quick and easy even for elaborate programs.

There should be a public display of the quality control charts. This gives the procedure acknowledged importance, encourages interest by personnel and visitors in high-quality work, and provides useful data for interpreting tests.

Out-of-Control Values

Depending on whether $\pm$ 3s or $\pm$ 2s limits are used, out-of-control values can be expected by chance alone once in 384 days or once in 22 days. What should be done when they occur?

1. For stable sample systems the first procedure is to repeat the analysis of the quality control material. At least half the time the second analysis will be in control, indicating some form of mishandling of the sample. One of the

commoner faults is failure to thaw out a frozen ampoule completely; because the heavier molecules settle out, the supernatant is not a true sample of the entire contents. If the new analysis is in control the batch is considered satisfactory and results of patient tests are released.

If the second analysis is out of control, all reports on patients are held up until the problem is identified and correct analyses can be performed.

2. For average of normal values or other systems using 95 percent confidence limits, a single out-of-control value leads to careful scrutiny of the procedure but does not usually require holding up patient results. If two days in close succession are out of control a thorough study is necessary.

3. A discrepancy between two systems—particularly stable samples and average of normal values—may occur, one being within proper limits and the other being out of control or consistently high or low although still in control. This may indicate the presence of a factor not common to both systems. Changes in blood-drawing techniques or patient diets, for example, will affect only the average of normal value samples. In one instance we found increased fasting blood glucose levels due to a new policy of giving all patients coffee with sugar on awakening; this kindly gesture affected our results measurably.

4. If a computer is in use, the out-of-control data may be gathered and decision strategy formulated as described in Chapter 17.

5. An out-of-control book is kept for entry of all out-of-control results. The entry should include the date, the cause of the problem as far as it can be elicited, and the measures taken to correct it.

6. What are the common causes of out-of-control values once improper sample thawing is excluded? The following list covers the majority of the problems we have encountered:

   a. New standards, differing in some way from those previously used.
   b. New reagents, improperly made up.
   c. Deterioration of reagents, particularly enzyme substrate. This usually gives warning by a progressive change of values before they actually appear out of control.
   d. Dirt in instrument tubing or aspirators. Apparently this often affects patient specimens and quality control serum before it affects standards used for calibration.
   e. Instrument malfunction of an erratic nature.

Sometimes the source of the problem cannot be identified. In this case it may be necessary to put in new standards, reagents, tubing, and so on in a massive "shotgun" attack.

Alarm Values
A useful tool for checking the quality of results which are sent out is two sets of "alarm" values which serve to initiate quick responses. One is for laboratory

use, to prevent ridiculous reports from being sent out. The other is for the attending physician, to alert him to a clinically dangerous situation verified by laboratory tests and demanding immediate attention. Every laboratory should have such lists.

The values for laboratory use comprise values so unlikely that they require checking before reporting. The rechecking involves first recalculation and check of decimal points; if the original result is confirmed, a new specimen should be drawn from the patient and analyzed. One common cause of these peculiar results is the drawing of blood from an intravenous tube into which an infusion is flowing; this should be avoided. If the two reports agree, the report is cleared with the supervisor and sent out. Not surprisingly, such unusual values occur most often when unusual tests are undertaken and the analyst is not familiar with the method or with the usual range of results. Examples of laboratory alarm values are: prothrombin time less than .75 or more than 5 times the control time, serum sodium under 100 mEq. per liter or over 170 mEq. per liter, serum calcium under 6 mg. per 100 ml.

The physician-list of alarm values indicates that the attending physician must be notified immediately of an unusual laboratory result so that he may undertake treatment promptly. Examples: serum glucose below 50 mg. per 100 ml. or above 350 mg. per 100 ml., serum bicarbonate below 10 mEq. per liter or above 40 mEq. per liter, serum sodium below 115 mEq. per liter or above 165 mEq. per liter, prothrombin time more than 3.5 times as long as the control time.

References

1. Amenta, J. S. Analysis of variance, control charts and the clinical laboratory: A system of quality control. Am. J. Clin. Pathol. 49:842–849, 1968.
2. Barnett, R. N., and Pinto, C. L. Evaluation of a system for precision control in the clinical laboratory. Am. J. Clin. Pathol. 48:243–247, 1967.
3. Bull, Brian S. "A Statistical Approach to Quality Control." In Quality Control in Haematology, edited by S. M. Lewis and J. F. Coster, pp. 111–121. London, New York, San Francisco: Academic Press, 1975.
4. Copeland, B. E. (Ed.). Quality Control Manual (rev. ed.). Chicago: American Society of Clinical Pathologists, 1967.
5. Dorsey, D. (Ed.). Manual for Workshop on Quality Control in Hematology. Chicago: American Society of Clinical Pathologists, 1964.
6. Hoffman, R. G., and Waid, M. E. The "average of normals" method of quality control. Am. J. Clin. Pathol. 43:134–141, 1965.
7. Hoffman, R. G., and Waid, M. E. Efficiency of the averages-of-normals method of laboratory quality control. Unpublished material, 1968.
8. Korpman, R. A., and Bull, B. S. The implementation of a robust estimator of the mean for quality control on a programmable calculator or a laboratory computer. Am. J. Clin. Pathol. 65:252–253, 1976.
9. Levey, S., and Jennings, E. R. The use of control charts in the clinical laboratory. Am. J. Clin. Pathol. 20:1059–1066, 1950.
10. Prangnell, P. R., and Johnson, P. H. A new method for quality control of the Coulter Model S. J. Clin. Pathol. 30:487–491, 1977.
11. Weinberg, M. S., and Barnett, R. N. Absence of analytic bias in a quality control program. Am. J. Clin. Pathol. 38:468–472, 1962.

11 Standardization

We have already indicated the need for standardization of laboratory reagents, pure chemicals, and equipment. In this chapter standardization is considered in more detail.

Chemical Standards

Radin [3] has written extensively on definitions and specifications of chemical standards. His section on the Primary Standard follows:

In the reference frame of usual analytical laboratory practice the primary standard is defined as a pure chemical substance that is used for the purpose of assaying a volumetric solution of unknown strength or for the preparation of a solution of known concentration. Although it is not always possible to select a substance for a primary standard with all the desired characteristics, it is generally stated that the primary standard should be selected with the following criteria in mind.

1. It must be a stable substance of definite composition.
2. It must be a substance that can be dried in the course of preparation, preferably at 105–110°, without change in composition.
3. It should have a high equivalent weight in order that weighing errors may have a relatively small effect.
4. It must be a substance that can be accurately analyzed.
5. Desired reactions should occur according to single, well-defined, rapid, and essentially complete processes.
6. The purity of a primary standard must be assured through well-defined qualitative tests of known sensitivity, or through preparation by a method that has been demonstrated to yield consistently a pure product, and by storage under conditions in which the product is entirely stable.

In almost every quantitative test, one of the first steps is to dissolve pure chemical in a solvent. This standard is then carried through the same analytic steps as the unknown sample, and calculations of the level in the unknown are made by comparison with those in the standard. If the pure material is not uniform or not what it is said to be, the levels of unknown will be determined incorrectly.

The great variation in hemoglobin levels in different laboratories and in different countries posed such a serious problem in 1954 that several U.S. agencies became involved in adopting a uniform method which could be standardized in an acceptable manner. At that time hemoglobin assays were supposed to be standardized in each laboratory by use of such indirect methods as iron content, oxygen binding, and so on. These methods were tedious and imprecise; there was not complete agreement on the conversion factors; the material assayed was not stable, so frequent reassays were necessary—but were rarely carried out. The ultimate solution to the problem was the adoption of the cyanmethemoglobin method with the use of a stable, readily produced standard, each batch of which is assayed by laboratories independent of the manufacturer. Batches meeting standard specifications are certified (in the United States by the Standards Laboratory of the College of American Pathologists [CAP]) and can then be purchased by individual laboratories to calibrate their own method [1].

Subsequently, standard specifications were drawn up for bilirubin and cholesterol, two materials of previously uncertain composition. The CAP presently certifies batches of bilirubin as meeting these specifications. The National Bureau of Standards (NBS) now produces a wide variety of certified pure chemicals for clinical laboratory standards. These are in most instances too expensive for daily use, but they provide a solid reference point with which commercially prepared pure materials can be compared.

Other materials useful in checking laboratory accuracy are the CAP Clinical Standard Solutions. Produced as ampouled primary standards (pure solutes in a pure matrix) these are then analyzed by three laboratories using a statistical scheme suggested by W. J. Youden and later published by Kambli and Barnett [2]. In essence, 12 paired analyses using the CAP materials are performed in parallel with 12 analyses using National Bureau of Standards Standard Reference Materials (SRM). Agreement must be within 1 percent or the paired t-test must indicate lack of significant disagreement between the two materials if the solutions are to be accepted.

Although the variability of most pure standards is not the major cause of interlaboratory differences, the existence of widely used pure material will provide the necessary backbone on which improvement of testing can be supported.

Serum Standards in Chemistry

Many of the large instruments that perform multiple types of analyses rely on a single preassayed material, either serum or a derivative, for calibration. The potential weakness of such a system is self-evident; if the "standard" material* does not contain the claimed amount of each constituent due to inaccurate analysis, deterioration, or any other factor, the results obtained will all be incorrect. The Food and Drug Administration is attempting to address the problem by developing a product class standard for such "calibrators" in which the manufacturer must state the exact values, the confidence limits within which these values fall, and the methods by which the values were derived. Meanwhile, the manufacturers are attempting to furnish similar data under the labelling provisions of the Medical Device legislation. Sometimes a calibrator cannot be assayed by conventional methods to yield "correct" results, yet it will work satisfactorily in the analytic system. Fortunately this is rare, because it poses a difficult dilemma in checking the results.

*Radin [3] proposes that the term *reference sample* or *reference serum* be used for these products.

One material which is serum-based and can be used as an excellent control material is the Survey Validated Serum available through the College of American Pathologists. Produced as extra vials with the survey materials, this can be purchased with a list of the results obtained by large numbers of participants using different specified methods. Many laboratories use this material to check their performance if questions arise concerning the accuracy of results. If one can obtain results close to the mean for the material, he can be confident that his general procedure is satisfactory.

Instrument Standards

Because most laboratory analyses are performed spectrophotometrically, it is apparent that the spectrophotometers themselves must be standardized and properly used. In this field the problem is not a lack of acceptable standards but failure to use them. Encouraging this failure is the usual analytic procedure whereby both standard and unknown material are subjected to the same process, so that the analyst assumes that instrumental errors will be canceled out—and often they are.

The instrument manufacturers contribute to this offhand attitude by their inexact claims for the performance of their devices. Almost inevitably an instrument is said to perform within ± 1 percent, with no further details. Realistically, performance should be defined at one or more specified wavelengths based on single determinations of the same material once a day in terms of standard deviation (or coefficient of variation) at a certain level of absorptivity. Furthermore, all the knobs should be reset between analyses. Actually, the manufacturers' claims are based all too often on a series of analyses, often of a blank, done one after another in a single run during which all the knobs were left in a fixed position. Naturally under these conditions, totally different from ordinary use, the precision is unrealistically good.

Parameters which can and should be checked are the following:

1. Wavelength settings at various levels, with necessary adjustments. For filter photometers, unsatisfactory filters should be discarded.
2. Absorptivity settings and performance.
3. Overall performance at different levels of absorptivity. Most instruments are linear in the center of the range (30% T. to 70% T.), but many are not linear near the ends of the range. The limits should be defined and the instrument used in the linear portion of the range.

In a long-term study of spectrophotometric performance [1], Copeland, King, and Willis present data from a seven-year, almost daily check of a Beckman DU Spectrophotometer. Using a U.S. National Bureau of Standards carbon yellow filter, they found for the seven years an average 3 CV of 0.5 percent, so that a genuine difference from month to month would be 0.5 percent; when such differences occurred they signified malfunction requiring repairs. Using a Chance neutral filter 0 N 10 for two years, the 3 CV was about

0.2 percent. The poorer performance with the carbon yellow occurs because the wavelength setting is critical, absorbance being measured at 540 nanometers on a sharply rising slope when absorption is plotted against wavelength. The Chance filter absorbance is not changed significantly by small changes in wavelength. It is apparent that an excellent spectrophotometer calibrated carefully and frequently is capable of excellent performance.

Unfortunately, most spectrophotometers and filter photometers do not exhibit this type of precision even when cared for adequately. Furthermore, these instruments are often used for long periods without any checking or servicing. To insure proper performance, frequent checks of wavelength setting, absorbance, and cleanliness of light-transmitting glass, as well as periodic changes of light bulbs, are necessary.

Overlapping

Whenever a new batch of reagent is to be introduced, it is wise to test a few patient samples using both the old and the new material. Five or 10 such comparison specimens are analyzed and the results compared. If the results are obviously identical or obviously widely divergent, no statistical analysis is needed; but if there is any doubt a paired *t*-test, as illustrated in Table 15-1, should be done.

This simple precaution often avoids a great deal of trouble.

References

1. Copeland, B. E., King, J., and Willis, C. The National Bureau of Standards' carbon yellow filter as a monitor for spectrophotometric performance: Successful experiences for 7 years in certifying the National Research Council's cyanmethemoglobin standard. *Am. J. Clin. Pathol.* 49:459–466, 1968.
2. Kambli, V. B., and Barnett, R. N. Control of accuracy of CAP clinical standards solutions. *Am. J. Clin. Pathol.* 61:912–915, 1974.
3. Radin, N. What is a standard? *Clin. Chem.* 13:55–76, 1967.

12 Duplicate Measurements

The routine performance of analyses in duplicate was at one time considered the best method for assuring the accuracy of results. It is still a useful procedure for tests involving certain difficult manipulations, such as extractions and washing precipitates, in which it is possible to lose a significant amount of material. If the duplicate results differ markedly, that is a clear indication to repeat the test. The duplicate analysis must start with separate aliquots of the original material and must be carried through all steps of the procedure. Merely reading the final result twice is not a true duplicate analysis.

Using the difference between duplicate readings as a measure of precision is useful only if the samples are carried through all the steps in parallel and also read at random in the run. If one is read immediately after the other, when all conditions affecting the instrument, the operator, and the environment are identical, the results will tend to be very close or identical, whereas day-to-day analyses may vary much more. If the procedure is basically inaccurate for any reason, the duplicate result will merely confirm the inaccurate value.

Another factor to be considered is operator bias. If the operator knows the first result, and if the second one is different, he tends to take a third reading "as a check"; most operators discard the second result if the third is closer to what is expected. Some supervisors insist that repeat readings be carried out until the desired closeness of results is achieved. This closeness of readings may be at an erroneous value accidentally achieved.

Much of the misunderstanding revolves around a statistical rather than an analytic concept. Statistically, it is more likely that the mean of several samplings will be close to the true mean than that any single sample will be close to the true mean. The pertinent formula is

$$SE = \frac{s}{\sqrt{n}}$$

In other words the standard error of a group of measurements is smaller than the standard deviation of single measurements by a factor equal to the square root of the number of measurements in the sample. If the true mean of a population is 20 and $s = 4$, then a single sample can be expected to be between 16 and 24 about 68 percent of the time; but if nine samples were taken, the SE of the average of the nine would be $\dfrac{4}{\sqrt{9}} = 1.33$, and averages between 16 and 24 would be expected 99.73 percent of the time.

When we apply this formula to repeat chemical analyses done at the same time by the identical technique, we find a sample whose value may be biased by foreknowledge of the expected result. More importantly, if the true content is 20 units but the analytic method is high by 4 units, the value obtained will be 24 units, and any number of repetitions will still yield results grouped around 24. For most tests, then, duplicate analyses do not help to assure accuracy but do waste lots of time.

Another aspect of duplicate measurements is the performance of two or more tests to study the same body function. The most familiar example is the determination of both hemoglobin and hematocrit on the same blood sample to check the accuracy of each against the other. Addison [1] found that in 560 such pairs there were only three disparate values, all the result of unusual fluid disturbances in severely burned patients, and even in these three cases the discrepancy had no clinical importance. This form of duplicate study provides no real check on accuracy and has no advantage over duplicates using a single form of measurement.

Known Versus "Blind" Duplicates

It is commonly found that if a known duplicate sample is analyzed, there is better agreement of the two samples than if a "blind" duplicate is tested in the same run. The assumption has always been that this result was related chiefly to foreknowledge of the expected value with resultant operator bias toward agreement of results. Weinberg and Barnett [2] studied this and found no such effect in analyses of a quality control sample whether introduced as a known or an unknown specimen. We concluded that the observed closeness of duplicates was due to physical closeness of the samples in the run and not to operator bias.

Operator bias may be important for tests involving a choice of readings, however, as compared to tests in which numerical readout or automation eliminates operator choice. Operator bias may also be encouraged by poor supervisory practices in which excessive reproducibility is demanded—beyond the capacity of the technique. For years medical students were taught that the five squares counted in an erythrocyte count must agree within 10 cells, or the whole count should be repeated. This is not possible because of the inherent sampling error, so the effect was to cause overt dishonesty rather than to produce accurate cell counts!

Use of truly blind duplicates does provide a useful index of reproducibility in actual practice, whereas use of known duplicates creates an erroneous impression of precision greater than is possible in patient samples analyzed from day to day.

References

1. Addison, S. J. Is routine ordering of both hemoglobin and hematocrit justifiable? *Can. Med. Assoc. J.* 95:974–975, 1966.
2. Weinberg, M. S., and Barnett, R. N. Absence of analytic bias in a quality control program. *Am. J. Clin. Pathol.* 38:468–472, 1962.

13 Detection of Laboratory Errors

We have already discussed quality control systems and survey samples, both useful in detecting either systematic or random errors. It is the latter which are the more difficult to detect and generally cause the most trouble. Some of the common problems follow.

Falsely Abnormal Values

If a test value is falsely and markedly abnormal, it is very likely to be repeated, either at once or during the course of treatment, and the discrepancy between the two values becomes obvious. Cumulative patient report forms make it easy to pick up discrepancies from day to day. Most clinicians faced with an abnormal test result that will lead directly to vigorous treatment take the precaution of repeating the test once or more often. This wise step serves to avoid catastrophes resulting from single random errors.

Falsely Normal Values

Falsely normal values are much more difficult to detect than abnormal ones because the tests are less likely to be repeated. An alert clinician may notice that the result does not fit the clinical picture, but for many tests this is impossible to detect. If the analysis is repeated for any reason the discrepancy becomes obvious.

Correct Value, Wrong Patient

The problem created by a value's being reported for the wrong patient is the same as that caused by one of the two errors just described. Every precaution should be taken to prevent these mix-ups.

Discordant Values

When a single physiologic function or constant is evaluated by two or more tests, random errors can sometimes be detected by comparison of the results. This requires a basic knowledge of pathophysiology. Typical examples follow.

Sodium 105 mEq. per liter, chloride 100 mEq. per liter, CO_2 25 mEq. per liter. Sodium must always exceed CO_2 plus chloride; therefore one of these three figures is wrong, probably the sodium.

BUN 5 mg. per 100 ml., creatinine 5 mg. per 100 ml. A low BUN could not accompany a high creatinine. One is wrong.

RBC 1.5 million per cubic millimeter, Hb 15 gm. per 100 ml. A very low erythrocyte count cannot accompany a normal hemoglobin level. Again, one value must be wrong.

Glucose tolerance test; fasting 200 mg. per 100 ml., ½ hour 80 mg., 1 hour 225 mg., 2 hour 300 mg., 3 hour 210 mg. This doesn't make sense. The subject appears to be diabetic, but how did the ½-hour value of 80 mg. appear? Are the first two values transposed? Is the discrepant value from the wrong patient? In any event, at least one of these values is wrong.

RBC 5.1 million per cubic millimeter on Monday, 3.0 million on Tuesday, 5.0 million on Wednesday. Either there was a sudden hemorrhage followed by transfusions, or the 3.0 million value is an error.

Delta Checks

By this term we mean checking differences for the same analyte between one analysis and the next, as in the RBC example just above. To use this as a laboratory tool for error detection the following procedures must be undertaken.

1. Instruct the computer to compare the results in a specified fashion, such as by comparing sequential samples, or the first one each day, or some other appropriate combination.
2. Decide what size difference is acceptable.
3. Have the computer identify values which exceed the acceptable difference and publish them in the desired way; also, hold up delivery of the report to the physician until it can be checked.
4. Develop a system for investigating these large differences. This system could involve automatic repetition of the second value, a phone call to the nursing station, a review of results by the pathologist, or study of the patient chart.

To date there are insufficient data on large-scale application of delta checks to portray their ultimate usefulness.

Single Values Outside Usual Limits

Values which are not compatible with life, or which are very rare, should always be checked. If the analytic data and calculations appear to be correct, a new sample should be drawn from the patient and a fresh analysis made.

Example: Serum chloride 20 mEq. per liter. This is not compatible with life but the patient is alive. The value is therefore wrong. A reasonable explanation is that the sample was drawn from tubing into which a solution of glucose in water was flowing.

Clinical Correlation

The modern clinician uses laboratory tests freely and develops a considerable skill in making clinical correlations with the results. He is in a good position to find random errors and report them to the laboratory personnel. Such reports are invaluable and demand immediate follow-up.

Less commonly, systematic errors may be suspected. In one published example [2] a systematic error in serum sodium was detected by the clinicians before the quality control systems were activated. (This was not so much an indictment of the systems as of the analytic technique; the acceptable limits were so wide as to be useless.) If a clinician feels that "all the hemoglobins are high," this is adequate reason for a careful reevaluation of the whole test procedure.

Frequency of Errors

The expected frequency of ordinary errors inherent in each method is known from the quality control studies. The frequency of large errors representing mistakes (outliers, in statistical terms) is very hard to calculate and varies greatly in different laboratories and different disciplines. A baseline figure of 1 in 2,000 analyses seems reasonable and is probably an irreducible minimum. Even computers and their operators probably do no better. Keeping mistakes to this minimum demands constant attention to every detail of procedure. The current great increase in testing inevitably increases the total number of errors. When an automated and computerized operation, totally divorced from patient care and clinician feedback, goes wrong, the outcome may be catastrophic; worst of all, it may be undetected for a long period. In one large laboratory I inspected, there was constant grumbling by the clinicians, who found many inexplicable and unreproducible results. It turned out (after a long time) that the computer periodically and erratically got "out of phase" with the samples; there might be 20 correct values but the next 20 would all be attributed to the wrong patients!

Error Rate and Choice of Methods

Some methods which work well in the research laboratory or under similar special conditions do not perform equally well in the field. As a general rule these are methods that involve difficult manipulations or numerous calculations. One good example is the Abell-Kendall [1] method for cholesterol. It is certainly the reference method and the most accurate; yet in surveys it usually is less precise than many other simpler methods that require fewer manipulations. This is one of many choices a laboratory director must make; shall he increase accuracy, knowing that he will thereby create more large random errors? Such decisions should be based on knowledge of the inherent character of the methods and of his organization's capability, as well as on the medical significance of his decisions.

References

1. Abell, L. L., Levy, B. B., Brodie, B. B., and Kendall, F. E. Simplified method for estimation of total cholesterol in serum and demonstration of its specificity. *J. Biol. Chem.* 195:357–366, 1952.
2. Van Peenen, H. S., and Lindberg, D. A. B. The limitations of laboratory quality control with reference to the "number plus" method. *Am. J. Clin. Pathol.* 44:322–330, 1965.

14 External Quality Control: Proficiency Surveys

The 1947 study of Belk and Sunderman [2] was a landmark in calling attention to the enormous variation in results achieved when different clinical laboratories examined the same specimens. The discrepancies were of such a magnitude that analysis of the same blood for glucose at two different hospital laboratories could have led to insulin administration at one and glucose administration at another!

Recognition of the problem and the urgent need to do something about it has led professional and governmental agencies into various programs whereby stable specimens are submitted to different laboratories for analysis. These may be used for education only, being followed by a technical critique; or they may be used to evaluate performance of individual laboratories and even for regulation of activities. The largest program, and the one with which I have been most closely connected, is that carried out by the Standards Committee of the College of American Pathologists (CAP); it is from this experience that most of the material in this section is derived.

Types of Materials

The most satisfactory material for surveys generally has been lyophilized serum. This is stable almost indefinitely, can be made in huge batches, and is easy to handle and easy to ship. It does require reconstitution, an extra step that may be a source of error. Liquid serum has been widely used in Australia [4] and apparently works well; it does not require reconstitution. In the U.S.A. problems have arisen with deterioration of liquid serum in the mails; creatinine, particularly, seems to be unstable because of its unstable equilibrium with creatine. Some stabilized cell samples for enumeration and hematocrit determination have worked well.

In the nonquantitative disciplines such as microbiology and cell morphology there are numerous problems of nomenclature, lack of uniformity of raw material, and so on. Identical color transparencies may be used for uniformity, even though they no longer simulate the usual laboratory specimens. Because these problems are not primarily statistical, we shall say no more about them.

Instructions

A critical factor in conducting a first-class survey is the preparation of clear, concise instructions for handling the specimen and reporting the results. Exact details of amount and type of diluent and how to add it must be given.

Equally important are instructions on how to fill in the questionnaire or

Table 14-1
Entries for Surveys
Circling Correct Values

Circle numbers already listed.

20	21	22	23	24	25	26	27	28	29
30	31	32	33	34	35	(36)	37	38	39
40	41	42	43	44	45	46	47	48	49

Table 14-2
Entries for Surveys
Filling in Boxes

Fill in blank spaces arranged as follows:

Vial C5 $\boxed{2}$ $\boxed{6}$ $\boxed{7}$· mg./100 ml.
whole numbers only

Vial C6 $\boxed{3}$ $\boxed{5}$ · $\boxed{2}$ mg./100 ml.
to 1st decimal place

report form, and this must be correlated with proper questionnaire design. Many mistakes are made in entering results, both in making actual numerical reports and in naming the method used. Acceptable forms provide for entries to be made in one of the two ways shown in Tables 14-1 and 14-2. Fewer incorrect entries occur when the method shown in Table 14-2 is employed.

METHODS. For many constituents there are only a few methods and their names are familiar to most participants; for other constituents, particularly enzymes, there are so many modifications of methods that accurate nomenclature is almost impossible at present.

Referee and Reference Laboratories

A good survey program requires the use of some sort of control laboratories. These were divided into two categories in the CLIA 1967 regulations (Title 42, part 74, subpart A, Sections 74.1 (j) and (k)) as published in the Federal Register Vol. 33, No. 253, Dec. 31, 1968. The categories were "referee" and "reference" defined as follows:

(j) A "referee" laboratory is a laboratory designated by the Secretary to examine specimens or other materials for purposes of proficiency testing using the same time schedule allowed for licensed laboratories and under conditions similar to those under which licensed laboratories examine materials.
(k) A "reference" laboratory is a laboratory designated by the Secretary to authenticate the identification, content, and titer of samples and other materials used or to be used in proficiency testing.

The role of the referees as designated is clear enough: They receive specimens in advance and send in their results, usually for analyses of several samples at daily intervals. The results are returned to the surveying agency to assure that the samples were stable and had the proper content of the constituent sought. If wide discrepancies are found between referees or between samples, something is wrong and the specimen cannot be used for a survey.

The role of the reference laboratory as defined by the National Communicable Disease Center is less clear. In principle it accepts the presumption that there is a "true" level for a given constituent, and that this level can be found by repeated very careful analysis. Unfortunately, for most biologic materials this is an unwarranted presumption. Most substances in body fluids are in some sort of equilibrium with others and each method of analysis disturbs this equilibrium in a different way; therefore there may be several "true" levels entirely dependent on the methods used.

After extensive experience the CAP Survey abandoned the reference laboratory concept for chemical analytes [3]. The participants' mean values were found to be more reliable in establishing the "true" values than were those of the reference laboratories.

Evaluation of Data

Effect of Methods

For reasons already discussed it is imperative that data first be classified by method of analysis. Certain methods give values definitely higher or lower than others. Separate statistical appraisal is made for each commonly used method. An example is shown in Table 14-3.

Note that three of the four commonly used methods give almost identical results, but the glucose oxidase is about 10 percent lower. If this method is considered acceptable, participants using it must be graded separately from those using the others. When methods are used by only a few participants, so that statistical evaluation is impractical, the mean for all standard methods is considered the applicable standard of performance.

Table 14-3
Survey Data*
Effect of Methods. Glucose (mg./100 ml.)

Method	Value
Somogyi-Nelson	234
Glucose oxidase	207
Ferricyanide AA	233
SMA 12	232

*CAP 1968 Comprehensive Survey Set C3, Vial C5.

Effect of Outliers and Their Elimination

In almost every survey there are one or more values which obviously reflect gross errors of transcription, decimal point, or unit of measurement. In fact the apparently poor results for calcium in some surveys are believed to include a considerable number reported in milliequivalents rather than milligrams, thereby halving the reported values. To eliminate these outliers, which cause a marked increase of the standard deviation and of the apparent ranges of performance, the CAP has proceeded in one of two directions:

1. Using all results, calculate $\bar{x}$ and $3s$ limits. Eliminate all values beyond $3s$. Recalculate $\bar{x}$ and s from the remaining values and again calculate $\bar{x}$ and $3s$. Eliminate all values beyond the new $3s$. Those values which still remain are now used to calculate statistics and acceptable limits.
2. Plot all values on a normal curve. Chop off any which by eye appear outside the curve. Calculate $\bar{x}$ and s from the remaining values.

An example of the effect of eliminating outliers is shown in Table 14-4. Note that after the 7 outliers in the right-hand column were removed the mean for the remaining 736 laboratories was changed only slightly (0.07), but the SD was cut to less than half (0.88 to 0.40). This changes the acceptable limits as follows:

Actual Limits	Adjusted Limits
1.88–5.40	2.77–4.37

Table 14-4
Survey Data
Effect of Eliminating Outliers. Phosphorus (mg./100 ml.)

Method	No. of Labs	Actual Mean	Actual s	Adjusted Mean	Adjusted s	Excluded Values
Phosphomolybdic acid	743	3.64	0.88	3.57	0.40	11.0, 12.9, 13.4, 6.9, 6.5, 13.2, 14.3

Acceptable Limits

After generating for each method the $\bar{x}$ and s values for all the participant results, it is necessary to set acceptable performance limits in some fashion. The 1977 CAP survey uses the following terms:

within $\pm 1s$	Good
not within $\pm 1s$ but within $\pm 2s$	Acceptable
outside $\pm 2s$	Not acceptable

Table 14-5
Survey Data
Computer Printout for Each Participant

1	2	3	4	5	6	7	8
Constituent	Specimen No.	Method	Participant's Result	Code*	Mean	Good Performance	Acceptable Performance
Glucose mg./100 ml.	CO5	Ferricyanide Auto-Analyzer	223	1	227	213–242	208–246
Creatinine mg./100 ml.	CO5	AutoAnalyzer	6.0†	1	5.5	5.0–5.9	4.8–6.1
Potassium mEq./L.	CO2	Flame Photometer	2.0‡	1	3.0	2.6–3.4	2.4–3.6
Alkaline phos. units	CO2	Bessey-Lowrey	19.0	10		See referee report	

*Code 1 means that the results are evaluated by participant values; 10 means that the method is not in common use and cannot be evaluated.
†Value acceptable; strive for good performance.
‡Value not acceptable.

These results appear on the computer printout as returned to the participant (Table 14-5).

Note that this system always considers almost 5 percent of values as unsatisfactory. If everyone performed equally well, each participant would expect about 1 in 20 values to be unsatisfactory, and officials who inspect the results should also expect this.

Another possible way to set limits is to use the referee values. This permits reporting performance back to the participants even before all the participant values are received. There are several drawbacks which prevent this system from being ideal, however.

1. There may be no referees available for methods widely used in small laboratories.
2. Referee limits may be wider than participant limits. This usually occurs when a single referee is systematically considerably different from the others.

Another problem is that of possible nonnormal distribution. In 1968 the CAP surveys were reanalyzed on the basis of percentiles, which do not assume a normal distribution, and the 95 percent limits set in this way were compared with those derived by the usual $\bar{x} \pm 2s$ limits. The only difference was for bilirubin in the very low range, about 0.4 mg. per 100 ml., the lower limits by percentiles being somewhat higher than those set by the normal distribution curve. It was believed that the normal distribution is therefore entirely acceptable for survey data of this type.

It is possible that at some future time an alternative plan such as limits of medical usefulness [1] might be employed to evaluate limits of good and acceptable performance. At this time, however, the best criterion seems to be "peer" performance as described here.

Youden Plots

In 1960 Youden [5] noted that in surveys of the kind described, wherein specimens are sent to a number of analysts, there was a great tendency for participants whose results were far from the others to shrug off the occurrence as an accident. This attitude did not lead to corrective action or improved performance. However, when two specimens were sent and the results were plotted as "Youden plots," it was apparent that most errors were systematic. Most analysts faced with two very low or two very high results would recognize that they were making a systematic error and would take action to correct the procedure. This form of plotting has been widely used by both the Australian [4] and American College of Pathologists. A representative example is illustrated in Figure 14-1.

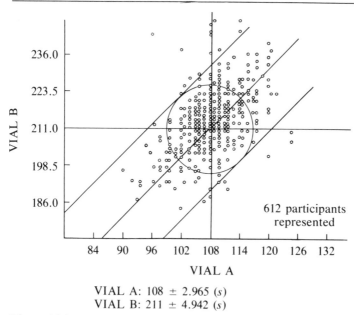

VIAL A: 108 ± 2.965 (s)
VIAL B: 211 ± 4.942 (s)

Figure 14-1
Youden plot for glucose survey (ferricyanide, AutoAnalyzer, mg./100 ml.). Each point represents value for one participant for the two samples A and B. Scale planned so that 1 unit = s horizontally or vertically. Horizontal line represents mean for all values for Vial B; vertical line represents mean for all values for Vial A. Circle is drawn at 3.035 s around junction of these lines. Oblique lines are 45° lines through center and at circumference of circle.

Table 14-6
Effect of Systematic Versus Random Variation

Performance	Expected Frequency		Actual Frequency	
	Number	Percent	Number	Percent
Good–Good	618.1	75.2	668	81.3
Good–Acceptable	124.9	15.2	52	6.3
Good–Not acceptable	64.1	7.8	47	5.7
Acceptable–Acceptable	6.6	0.8	11	1.3
Acceptable–Not acceptable	6.6	0.8	15	1.8
Not acceptable–Not acceptable	1.6	0.2	29	3.5
Total	822	100	822	99.9

Within the circle there is a reasonably even distribution of points, with some paucity on the edge of the left upper and right lower quadrants. However, note that outside the circle almost all the points are in the left lower and right upper quadrants, i.e., the participants found both values lower or higher than they should be. This indicates the overwhelming importance of systematic as opposed to random error. Youden [6] calculated for one of these surveys what the participant results indicated. Each value was called "good" if within $1.5s$ of the mean, "acceptable" if more than $1.5s$ but less than $2s$ from the mean, and "not acceptable" if more than $2s$ from the mean. For each value, then, 86.6 percent should have been good, 8.8 percent acceptable, and 4.5 percent not acceptable. Youden tabulated the expected and observed frequency of each combination as presented in Table 14-6. Note that the good–good category is *better* than expected by 6 percent, and the not acceptable–not acceptable is *worse* by 3.3 percent, values being 17.5 times as numerous as expected! The last figure is particularly enlightening in pinpointing the systematic nature of truly poor laboratory results.

A somewhat unexpected finding from the CAP survey [3] was the existence of three variables of approximately equal size, rather than just those of simple precision and accuracy. By comparing samples sent out as unknown pairs at a single time with samples sent out as unknown pairs several months apart, Gilbert [3] found that within-run precision, long-term precision, and accuracy are all important in explaining interlaboratory variability. The long-term precision factor has not been satisfactorily explained as yet; the others are apparent, and their solution, if necessary, is well understood.

Effect of Surveys

It has been extremely difficult to decide whether proficiency surveys have accomplished their goal of improving performance. This is due in part to

Table 14-7
Improvement in Laboratory Performance between 1949 and 1969*

Constituent	Coefficient of Variation	
	1949 (aqueous)	1969 (serum)
Glucose	16.3	8.0
Urea N	64	13
Chloride	16.4	5.2
Calcium	28	11
Cholesterol	24	19

*CAP surveys.

changes in methods of evaluating the results, but in much greater part to changes in the participants surveyed. Specifically, if we start with 50 laboratories which improve each year, but we add 50 new participants each year, the effect of the new entries will obscure the changes in the original members. Furthermore, there have been a myriad of improvements in laboratory testing in recent years, so that better performance cannot necessarily be attributed to surveys. Table 14-7 indicates that there had been a significant improvement in the years 1949–69. Both columns represent CAP surveys calculated the same way. The 1949 survey used aqueous samples, and the 1969 survey used serum samples which offer greater problems in analysis, so the true change is even greater than that indicated.

A follow-up study by Gilbert [3] demonstrated improving precision for 10 analytes determined in each annual CAP survey from 1969 through 1975, as indicated in Table 14-8.

Interlaboratory Variability

It follows from what has been said about surveys that differences between results from different laboratories are more commonly systematic than random. If we accept this concept there are several corollaries.

NORMAL VALUES. If each laboratory reported its own normal values and expressed patient results in the context of its own normal values (see Chapter 9), a physician dealing with results from different centers could handle them more easily. Unfortunately, there are different methods and many pitfalls in calculating these normal values. Furthermore, exact numerical results are necessary

Table 14-8*
Overall Precision, Comprehensive Chemistry Survey
Expressed as CV (%)†

| | Coefficient of Variation | |
	1969	1975
Calcium	7.8	3.6
Glucose	7.0	7.7
Potassium	6.3	2.3
Sodium	3.2	1.4
Urea	13.7	6.3
Uric acid	10.7	6.6
Chloride	4.5	2.2
Creatinine	16.5	10.4
Phosphorus	11.5	7.0
Total protein	6.6	3.4

*Data abstracted from Gilbert [3], Tables V and VI, p. 68.
†All serum-based material.
Note that glucose has not improved for reasons not presently clear. Many of the others cannot be improved much further with current methodology.

for patient care in some instances, as in the case of electrolyte balance, as well as for comparison with the usual published values.

METHODS. Some of these systematic differences result from the use of methods which are basically different. If everyone used the same method this source of differences should vanish, but the resultant straitjacket of conformity would cripple laboratory progress. Anyone who has dealt with methods prescribed or supported by official agencies can bear witness to the difficulty, often the impossibility, of altering these methods even after they are shown to be archaic or totally incorrect. Many considerations other than uniformity enter into choice of methods in varying contexts of patient care and laboratory needs. (See Chapters 15 and 19.) Survey results can and should be used for recommendations as to acceptability of methods. Certain methods consistently yield erratic results or mean values substantially different from all others, whereas some just as consistently provide good precision and mean values similar to those for all methods. Use of obviously poor methods should be discouraged, and use of good methods judged by survey results should be encouraged. Other factors of convenience and accuracy must also be considered, but the methods that perform the best in the field are often those which are also the most convenient.

Recent CAP surveys made use of a unique method to compare "true" values to the mean of participants [3]. The National Bureau of Standards measured certain survey specimen analytes using a so-called definitive method (in this case a double-isotope dilution–mass spectrometry method), one which appears to give exactly correct results as far as present scientific methods permit. For calcium, the participant values (eight specimens) ranged from 0.3 percent to 2.6 percent lower than NBS when all methods were averaged; the average was 1.3 percent low. For individual selected methods, the averages ranged from identical to 1.5 percent low. For potassium, the participant levels averaged 0.8 percent higher than NBS values for all methods.

Although similar studies have not been published for other constituents, there is no reason to believe that they would differ. This is excellent evidence that for at least some constituents the mean of participants is a very close approximation to the truth.

STANDARDIZATION. Within each method, and indeed for all methods, there are numerous areas where standardization of material and instruments can greatly reduce systematic errors. This represents a fertile field for both technical and statistical study and one with great promise for future narrowing of interlaboratory variation.

Using Survey Results in the Individual Laboratory

When the printout from a survey arrives, the laboratory director scrutinizes it promptly for values that are good, acceptable, or not acceptable. Those which are not good call for further investigation. After excluding transcription and transposition errors, the important question is whether the poor values (if any) are random or systematic. Results of a single survey consisting of two samples may answer this at once. Table 14-9 shows such results. Here the values are obviously high on both ampoules, well outside the $2s$ or even the $3s$ level for the group; the need for immediate action is obvious. Sometimes the values are acceptable but are both high or low, suggesting systematic bias. This should be followed up by observing the values of the next survey.

At the end of the year eight samples for each constituent have been received. It is very worthwhile to analyze all eight for closeness to the mean. From the eight differences one can calculate mean difference and s of the differences and do a t test to determine whether there is a statistically significant bias. Table 14-10 shows an example of such calculations. The significant 5 percent value for 7 df is 2.365. The value of 2.847 exceeds this; calcium values are definitely low for the year and action is necessary.

If each laboratory would check its performance this way there would soon be

Table 14-9
Survey Results Indicating Need for Immediate Action

Constituent	Participant's Result	Code†	Mean	Acceptable
Glucose X1	120*	1	97.1	87.0–107.2
Glucose X2	163*	1	143.2	131.2–155.2

*Not acceptable.
†Code 1 means that the results are evaluated by participant values.

Table 14-10
Survey Results
t Test on 8 Samples for a Year Indicates Systematic Error
Calcium (mg./100 ml.)

Sample	Participant's Value	Survey Mean	Difference	Difference Minus Bias	$\left(\dfrac{\text{Difference}}{\text{Minus Bias}}\right)^2$
01	8.0	8.2	−0.2	+ .1	.01
02	10.7	11.3	−0.6	− .3	.09
03	7.4	7.4	0	+ .3	.09
04	9.5	9.9	−0.4	− .1	.01
05	10.2	10.1	+0.1	+ .4	.16
06	12.5	13.3	−0.8	− .5	.25
07	8.5	8.7	−0.2	+ .1	.01
08	10.3	10.6	−0.3	0	0
			$\Sigma = -2.4$		$\Sigma d^2 = .62$
			$\bar{x}_d = -0.3$		

$$s = \sqrt{\frac{\Sigma d^2}{n-1}} = \sqrt{\frac{.62}{7}} = \qquad .298$$

$$t = \frac{\text{diff } \sqrt{n}}{s} = \frac{.3\sqrt{8}}{.298} = \qquad 2.847$$

much greater uniformity of results. The same sort of procedure is being undertaken in several states by use of identical quality control material for many laboratories. This permits comparison of the mean values of all participants with those of each individual laboratory on a continuing basis; thus each director soon learns if his values are low, high, or median with respect to the group.

References

1. Barnett, R. N. Medical significance of laboratory results. *Am. J. Clin. Pathol.* 50:671–676, 1968.
2. Belk, W. P., and Sunderman, F. W. A survey of the accuracy of chemical analyses in clinical laboratories. *Am. J. Clin. Pathol.* 17:853–861, 1947.
3. Gilbert, R. K. CAP "Interlaboratory Survey Data and Analytic Goals." In *Proceedings of CAP Aspen Chemistry Conference, 1976.* Skokie, Ill.: College of American Pathologists, 1977.
4. Hendry, P. I. A. *College of Pathologists of Australia: Report of Scientific Meetings No. 3, August 1963, and No. 4, August 1964.* Sydney: College of Australian Pathologists, 1964.
5. Youden, W. J. The sample, the procedure and the laboratory. *Anal. Chem.* 32:23A–37A, 1960.
6. Youden, W. J. Personal communication, 1969.

15 Choice of Methods

The choice of methods for use in the clinical laboratory is governed by many considerations. These include accuracy, precision, tendency to large random errors, convenience, expense, availability of equipment, availability of personnel, rapidity of performance, and use to which the information will be put. The rapid proliferation of "kits" as well as automated instruments has created so many alternatives for the laboratory director that he often feels bewildered. In this chapter some aspects of making these choices are discussed.

General Principles

FIELD TRIAL. No major device or system should ever be purchased unless it can first be tried out for at least a week in the laboratory. Any reputable vendor will be glad to permit a field trial.

OBSERVATION IN USE. If a large or expensive device is being considered, it should first be watched in operation somewhere, preferably in a laboratory similar to the one in which its use is being considered. It may be obvious at once that it takes more space or utilities or special conditions than can be furnished. It may create heat, odors, or noise which cannot be coped with.

COST ESTIMATES. At least preliminary calculations should be done of the cost per test, based on the volume of the laboratory in which the device will be used. Many embarrassing and annoying miscalculations, partly engendered by high-pressure marketing tactics, have occurred.

OPERATOR. A series of planned tests should be carried out by a specific person assigned to try out the device. All too often the director chooses a competent but excessively busy technologist and says, "Here, try this!" In any large laboratory there should be one or more individuals primarily assigned to "research and development" work. Even in a small laboratory some personnel time must be assigned for this function.

ADEQUATE TIME. When a field trial is performed, adequate time must be allowed to familiarize the operator with the technique before data is collected. If the manufacturer's representative has time to assist for a day or more, this helps assure that the instrument is performing as well as possible.

Comparing Tests

Usually a new method is being considered to replace one already in use. The new one is said to be cheaper, easier, quicker, or better in some other way. If the present method provides adequate accuracy and precision as judged by prior performance, the new and old methods can then be compared directly on patient specimens. If the present method is not considered a good one, other types of tests must be conducted.

Patient Comparison Data

For ordinary quantitative tests (e.g., glucose, BUN) 40 patient samples should be analyzed, preferably not more than 5 day. If the tests are done in a shorter time span, reagent or instrument deterioration may be overlooked. It is imperative that the patient samples include sufficient examples of each clinically important range—low, normal, and high. This may require preselection of samples. Each specimen is analyzed by both old and new methods, with due precaution to avoid sample spoilage. The data is collected on a form as illustrated in Table 15-1. In this table 10 values have been used instead of 40 for purposes of illustration only.

After the values in columns 1, 2, 3, and 4 are entered, calculations are undertaken. The values in column 3 are added and then divided by n (in this

Table 15-1
Comparison of Methods
Blood Glucose (mg./100 ml.)

Col. 1	Col. 2	Col. 3	Col. 4	Col. 5	Col. 6	Col. 7
Specimen No.	Date	Result: Old Method	Result: New Method	Difference (R − T)*	Difference Minus Bias	Col.6 Squared
1	29	76	74	2.0	−7.6	57.76
2	29	197	189	8.0	−1.6	2.56
3	29	92	76	16.0	6.4	40.96
4	29	108	100	8.0	−1.6	2.56
5	29	189	186	3.0	−6.6	43.56
6	30	107	100	7.0	−2.6	6.76
7	30	98	81	17.0	7.4	54.76
8	30	104	92	12.0	2.4	5.76
9	30	91	77	14.0	4.4	19.36
10	30	121	112	9.0	−0.6	0.36
		$\Sigma = 1{,}183$	1,087			234.40
		$\bar{x} = 118.3$	108.7			

bias $(\bar{d}) = 9.6$

$$s_d = \sqrt{\frac{\Sigma(d - \bar{d})^2}{n - 1}} = \sqrt{\frac{234.40}{9}} = \sqrt{26.044} = 5.10$$

Reference (old method) result minus *test* (new method) result.

case 10) to find the mean. Column 4 is handled similarly. The difference (old minus new mean) is the bias, or mean difference, or $\bar{d}$, in this example 9.6. Column 5 values are found by subtracting each test value from the corresponding old method value. Column 6 is found by subtracting the bias from each value in column 5. (If the bias were a negative figure it would be *added* to the column 5 values.) Column 7 values are the column 6 values squared.

To find the standard deviation of the difference the formula is

$$s_d = \sqrt{\frac{\Sigma(d - \bar{d})^2}{n - 1}}$$

Finally a *t* test is performed using the formula

$$t = \frac{\bar{d} \sqrt{n}}{s_d} = \frac{9.6 \sqrt{10}}{5.10} = \frac{9.6 \times 3.1623}{5.10} = \frac{30.358}{5.10} = 5.95$$

This *t* value exceeds the significant value for 9 df, 5 percent probability, of 2.262.

We now know that the new method averages 9.6 mg. lower than the old, and that this is statistically significant. We also know that *s* of the difference, *after correcting for the bias*, is 5.10 mg.; in other words the two values would differ from each other by 5.10 mg. or less 68 percent of the time after the 9.6 mg. bias was subtracted from the old method. A bias of this size is undesirable but could be handled by the physician once he was made aware of it. The agreement of the two methods after this correction is reasonably close.

Before carrying out these calculations it is first advisable to rearrange the data in Table 15-1, in order of ascending values of the old method, from lowest to highest. After this is done, the corresponding values are entered in columns 4 and 5. If the column 5 values appear significantly different in the low range from those in the middle or high range, it is proper to divide the series into two or three levels (not more) and to calculate each group separately. We might find, for instance, that the new method values were high in the high range only, and this might not create any problems in medical practice.

An additional step which is useful is to graph the results. Each sample result is plotted as a single point, the new method values on the vertical axis and the old method values on the horizontal axis (Figure 15-1). Ideally all points should fall on a 45° axis going through the left lower corner. Shift away from the corner is due to systematic bias; shift away from a 45° line indicates a discrepancy at different levels.

To recapitulate this portion of the procedure: We collect 40 patient samples, preferably over eight days, analyze by the old and new methods, rearrange in ascending order to determine the need for subdividing the 40 values, calculate bias and *s* of difference on all 40 tests or the necessary subdivisions, and make use of a *t* test to determine whether the bias is significant.

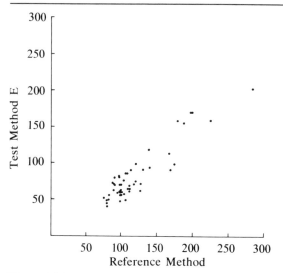

Figure 15-1
Graph of results when a reference and a test glucose (mg./100 ml.) method were compared on 50 patient samples. By "eye fit" it can be seen that there is some systematic bias, the reference values being somewhat higher. Spread of points away from a 45° line is excessive, so erratic performance is also evident. (From Barnett and Youden [4].) © 1970, J.B. Lippincott Co.

Further Tests

So far we have assumed that we have prior data on the old method and are satisfied with it. Such data might include quality control pool studies to establish the precision and survey results to indicate the accuracy of the method.

Suppose we were not satisfied with our existing method or had too little information about it. This situation arose commonly when we undertook studies of commercial kits [1–4], and we had to know the performance of the reference method in the hands of the laboratory carrying out the analyses. The available techniques include reproducibility studies and recovery experiments.

Reproducibility Studies

Originally, reproducibility studies were set up for pure aqueous solutions whose levels were low, medium, and high relative to the usual clinical levels. This assured accuracy because such solutions, made up from very pure chemicals, were of known composition. Unfortunately, it became obvious in our study of glucose kits that reagent systems which were satisfactorily accurate and precise for the analysis of pure aqueous solutions were sometimes totally unsatisfactory for use in such complex mixtures as blood serum. Table 15-2 gives some examples. Assuming the reference method values are correct, E and F produce reasonable results for the aqueous solutions but are both

Table 15-2
Aqueous Versus Serum CV (Expressed in mg./100 ml. as $\bar{x} \pm 1$ CV)

Method	Aqueous	Serum
Reference	90.2 ± 3.21	89.4 ± 8.06
E	84.2 ± 2.29	58.6 ± 22.11
F	88.0 ± 6.96	76.1 ± 22.73
R	88.2 ± 5.06	84.2 ± 4.14

inaccurate and imprecise when tested with serum. On the other hand, R gives results which are similar in aqueous solutions and serum.

It is therefore more realistic to use serum pools for the reproducibility studies. Securing or preparing these pools may be difficult. Frozen pooled serum as used in some quality control program, is suitable for at least one level. Another source is abnormal human serum, which can be used as collected and preserved or can be mixed with normal human serum. Lyophilized material as commercially prepared is also useful. When commercial material is used the following precautions should be observed:

1. Buy enough of one lot number to carry out the whole experiment.
2. Use the assay value, if any, as a guide, not as a target value.
3. Some commercial materials are of animal origin or are "spiked" with animal enzymes. They may give erroneous results in methods designed for use on human sera.

Once material is selected it should be analyzed once a day for 20 days. If a suitable reference method is available the results should be tabulated and calculated exactly as the patient comparison studies (pp. 134–135). In addition, the standard deviation for each method should be calculated using either of the usual formulas:

$$s = \sqrt{\frac{\Sigma(x - \bar{x})^2}{n - 1}} \quad \text{or} \quad s = \sqrt{\frac{\Sigma x^2 - \dfrac{(\Sigma x)^2}{n}}{n - 1}}$$

At each level chosen, then, we have calculated $\bar{x}$ and s of the difference. We can do an F test with the s for each method, and we can decide if there is a significant bias by the t test with the formula

$$t = \frac{\text{bias } \sqrt{n}}{s_d}$$

n being 20.

In addition to t-test statistics, the linear regression calculations described in Chapter 6 are often useful. In our own programs the computer performs all of these calculations and prints out the results.

Sometimes in evaluating a technique no reference method is available locally. Specimens can be mailed to reference laboratories if the ingredient to be determined is stable, and the results entered exactly as if they had been determined locally.

Recovery Experiments

If there is no reference method, then the material is analyzed by the test method only to derive the s. The accuracy of the method must be found by collateral methods such as other chemical or physical techniques. In addition, the recovery experiment is useful. In experiments of this type a base material is spiked by adding known amounts of the pure chemical for which analysis is desired. The base and the spiked materials are then subjected to analysis by both reference and test methods.

In the College of American Pathologists' protocol enough pure chemical is added to raise the levels by approximately 20 percent, 50 percent, and 100 percent of normal levels. In our glucose study [2] we found the base level of the serum pool to be 84 mg. per 100 ml. We therefore wished to raise it by 16.8 mg. (20%), 42 mg. (50%), and 84 mg. (100%). This procedure is carried out as follows. We make up a concentrated aqueous solution of glucose, 400 mg. per 100 ml., by dissolving 400 mg. of glucose in 0.2 percent benzoic acid solution and diluting to a final volume of 100 ml. with water. (The benzoic acid is used to preserve the glucose.) The calculation to make 100 ml. of material whose glucose level is 126 mg. per 100 ml. (84 mg. base + 42 added) follows: Let y = ml. of 400 mg. per 100 ml. glucose solution. Then

$$100 - y = \text{ml. of 84 mg. per 100 ml. base material}$$
$$400y + 84 \, (100 - y) = 100 \times 126$$
$$316y = 4{,}200$$
$$y = 13.29 \text{ ml.}$$
$$100 - y = 86.71 \text{ ml.}$$

Therefore we add 13.29 ml. of the 400 mg. per 100 ml. glucose solution to 86.71 ml. of base material. Similar calculations are carried out for the other levels.

We now analyze in a single run the base material and the three spiked samples by both methods, or by the test method only if there is no reference method, performing each analysis in triplicate. The data are tabulated as shown in columns 1 and 2 of Table 15-3.

Calculations are then carried out. Add the figures in column 1, yielding 4P + 142.8, representing the pool value (P) by the test method. Add the figures in column 2, yielding 382.6. Calculate P by the formula 4P = 382.6 minus 142.8; P = 60.0. This estimate of P is based on 12 analyses and is therefore more accurate than the 67.0 based on 3 analyses.

Table 15-3
Recovery Studies: Glucose (mg./100 ml.)

Col. 1 Sample	Col. 2 Values Found*	Col. 3 Recovery	Col. 4 Difference from Actual	Col. 5 Allowed Difference
A P†	67.0	—	—	—
B P + 16.8	82.3	22.3	5.5	9.18
C P + 42.0	102.3	42.3	0.3	9.18
D P + 84.0	131.0	71.0	13.0	11.09
4P + 142.8	382.6			

*Average of triplicate analyses.
†Serum pool.

Column 3 is then found by subtracting P (60.0) from each of the values in column 2. Column 4 values are differences between the recovery values in column 3 and the amount known to have been added as recorded in column 1.

The allowed difference in column 5 is calculated from the serum pool reproducibility studies at the level nearest that in column 2. At this level s is found and divided by 1.732 (the square root of 3) because analysis was done in triplicate; the result is multiplied by 2 because we seek $2s$ limits. In our example the pool level of 89.5 was the one nearest to the column 2 values for lines B and C; s at 89.5 is 7.95; divided by 1.732 is 4.59; multiplied by 2 is 9.18.

The next higher serum pool value was 184.3, and s is 11.73 at that level. By linear interpolation between 89.5 and 184.3, s at 131 is 9.60, divided by 1.732 is 5.54, multiplied by 2 is 11.08.

When we compare the allowed differences in the table with those found in column 4, lines B and C are acceptable, line D is not. We can therefore conclude that this method does not produce satisfactory recovery of glucose in the higher range.

When they are applicable, recovery studies are relatively quick and reliable guides to accuracy. It may not be possible to find pure materials, or if available they may not be soluble in diluents compatible with body fluids.

Interference Studies

Certain methods are susceptible to interference by analytes other than the one being tested. For example, many older cholesterol methods give falsely high values when the serum bilirubin is elevated. This sort of interference is documented by adding known final concentrations of the suspected interfering substance to several patient sera, then analyzing these sera with and without the additive.

For example, we wish to decide whether bilirubin at levels of 5 and 10 mg./dl. interferes with cholesterol determination so we add it to serum in the dilutions shown in Table 15-4.

Table 15-4
Addition of Bilirubin Sol. and Sodium Carbonate to Serum

	Dilutions		
	Serum. ml.	Bilirubin Sol. ml.	Sodium Carbonate. ml.
5 mg.	.875	.125	0
Control	.875	0	.125
10 mg.	.750	.250	0
Control	.750	0	.250

Table 15-5
Cholesterol Values (mg./dl)

Patient	1	2	3	4	5	$\bar{x}$
5 mg. bilirubin	120	230	180	310	240	216.0
Control	115	235	165	290	220	205.0
10 mg. bilirubin	125	235	190	300	225	215.0
Control	98	202	155	266	206	185.4

We therefore make similar dilutions for five patient sera and analyze the four samples from each patient for cholesterol. The results are given in Table 15-5.

We observe increases of 11 mg. above the control at the 5 mg. bilirubin level and 29.6 mg. above the control at the 10 mg. bilirubin level. Are these significant? We calculate the s_d at each level and then enter this into the formula

$$t = \frac{\text{diff } \sqrt{n}}{s_d}$$

At the 5 mg. level $s_d = 10.8$ and $t = 2.27$ and at the 10 mg. level $s_d = 6.69$ and $t = 9.89$. For 4 df the critical level of t at the 5 percent level is 2.776. Therefore we have not established that 5 mg. of bilirubin creates a definite interference, but we can be quite confident that 10 mg. does.

Enzymes

It is very difficult to perform comparisons of tests for enzymes. Enzyme units are entirely method-related and depend on specific substrates, direction of reaction, concentration of reagents, pH, and temperature, among other variables. Furthermore, enzymes of animal and human origin may behave very differently. Pure enzymes for recovery or accuracy studies are not available. It is unrealistic to expect different methods to be related in a linear fashion at different levels of concentration. Table 15-6 illustrates this with the ratio of

Table 15-6
Enzyme Method Comparison
Alkaline Phosphatase*

Method	Ratio
Bodansky	5.49
King-Armstrong	20.61
Bessey-Lowrey	34.73
Babson-Read	142.68

*CAP survey 1-3-67.

alkaline phosphatase values for the high level ampoule to those for the normal level ampoule for the CAP Chemistry Survey 1-3-67 for several methods frequently used.

Fortunately most laboratories can distinguish low, normal, and elevated values for the enzymes commonly studied, with sufficient accuracy for medical uses.

When enzyme methods are to be evaluated the following procedures are recommended:

1. Reproducibility studies using commercially prepared lyophilized material at normal and at one or more high levels. Calculate s as CV rather than in units. Perform once-a-day analyses for 20 days. Carry out in parallel with existing method or other reference method if possible.
2. Patient comparison studies for 40 patients. Make a graph indicating one point for each patient. Attempt to keep the scales for the reference and test methods approximately proportional. Draw perpendicular lines to separate normal from abnormal values if they are available. This will show vividly whether both methods indicate normal, low, and high on the same samples.

Precautions to Follow in Method Comparison Studies

In order to be suitable for statistical analysis, studies of this sort must be carefully planned in advance. In comparing a reference method to a test method, neither should suffer from a bias introduced by the experimental technique. We have evolved certain procedures from experience with many studies in this field, particularly one of GOT kits [4], and these are detailed below:

1. The reference method should be chosen with great care, based on suitable literature references, consultation with experts, and (if possible) the personal experience of the investigator. Results are more reproducible if an automated method can be used. One good source of information is the CAP survey material. For example, Table 15-7 shows an adapted segment of the creatinine results obtained in the 1974 survey [6].

Method A would obviously be excellent, whereas Method C has a large bias and poor precision and would be unacceptable. The manual comparative

Table 15-7
Creatinine Methods

Method	Precision within Lab (%)	Inaccuracy (Average %)
Manual (comparative)	12.3	0
Automated		
Method A	6.8	− 1.4
Method B	8.4	− 6.5
Method C	38.8	+22.4
Mean level is 1.20 mg./dl.		

Adapted from Gilbert [6].

method is considered absolutely accurate but is much less precise than either automated method A or B.

It is also likely that a specific reference method will achieve official sanction for FDA use in the future, and that it will presumably be acceptable to the laboratory community at large. Such a method might be practical for routine use; but even if it were not, it would serve to provide a baseline against which all other methods would be tested.

During the evaluation the reference method must be monitored as closely as the test method to assure its continuing performance at the expected level. This involves carrying out precision studies simultaneously by both test and reference methods.

2. The entire analytic portion of the experiment should be completed in as short a time as possible, rarely to exceed 60 days. This is necessary to avoid the effects of long-time cyclical within-laboratory variation which Gilbert [6] has described in analyzing CAP survey data.

3. Enough control material should be obtained to carry out the entire project and to provide a considerable excess in case repetitive analyses are needed. Precautions to avoid deterioration after reconstitution are important. Ordinarily, reconstituted materials should be kept refrigerated and used the day of preparation.

4. Enough reagents should be obtained for the entire project if feasible. If there is a need to study different lots this can be done by proper designing of the original protocol and by subsequent analysis of variance (ANOVA). For example, if we wish to study two lots (1 and 2) that are allegedly similar and that have a long shelf-life, we can alternate their use but also introduce enough randomization to avoid possible problem patterns (see Chapter 7, Randomization). If we use lot 1 for the first half and lot 2 for the second half of the experiment, we might confuse the effect of the lots with that of deterioration of reagents. In our GOT study [4] we found lot variability for enzyme reagents at the high level but not at the normal level in two of eight lots of 4 products analyzed on the broad

band-pass spectrophotometer and for 2 of 17 products when the narrow band-pass instrument was employed. This is an excellent example of a complex interaction involving the material analyzed, the instrument, the level of analyte, and the reagent lot.

5. The number and level of patient samples must be decided in advance. For some tests very low or very high levels may not be suitable for comparison; conversely, selection of only normal specimens may hide the inability of a method to identify the abnormals. Particularly in comparison of methods for enzyme analysis, very high levels may not be comparable because of difference in the rate of substrate exhaustion. In our GOT study we avoided samples higher than six times the upper limit of normal by the reference method.

6. All the analytic instruments must be checked regularly. For example, spectrophotometers should be monitored frequently for wavelength accuracy with a didymium or holmium oxide filter, and for absorbance linearity with neutral density filters.

7. To avoid spoilage, expiration dates must not be exceeded; leftover reagents should be discarded if the instructions so indicate. Patient samples must be handled appropriately, usually by prompt analysis, or by prompt separation of serum or plasma followed by refrigeration or freezing. If there is inadequate published data it may be necessary to validate the method used to preserve the samples. For example, we demonstrated by ANOVA [4] that GOT values did not change in 20 days in a comparison of 84 samples examined first fresh and later after freezing.

8. The order in which the two methods are carried out should assure that no opportunity for bias is introduced. If samples can be analyzed simultaneously by the two or more methods being compared, this is fine; however, it may mean that we are also comparing two different technologists as well as the two methods. If one person is carrying out work with both methods, he should alternate the order of testing; for example, we applied the test method (T) first on alternate days 1–10, then the reference method (R) first on alternate days 11–20:

Day	1	2	3	4	5	6	7	8	9	10	11	12	13	14	15	16	17	18	19	20
Done First	T	R	T	R	T	R	T	R	T	R	R	T	R	T	R	T	R	T	R	T

The comparative analyses should be done on the same day (or days).

9. The analysts must have adequate time to try out the methods and to verify their performance before a formal protocol is started. Repeated analyses of single samples or pools by both methods will establish whether the desired proficiency has been achieved. If manufacturers' representatives ordinarily provide instruction, this must be arranged. Directions are to be followed *exactly* as written, even if they appear incorrect. If the directions were adequate we found that two skilled technologists obtained identical results [4]: this was tested by ANOVA as described in Chapter 5, Problem 1.

10. Decisions about "outliers" in the reproducibility studies should be made in advance. Ordinarily, one obvious outlier in 20 day-to-day analyses can be summarily discarded; but if there seem to be two or more that are not explained by known procedural error, all values should be retained for calculations.

11. If possible, readings should be taken and recorded as they are obtained, but calculations should be avoided until the day's work is done. This helps insure an absence of operator bias in which the analyst takes "one more reading" because he "knows" the first one is wrong! Some analysts subconsciously hope a method will succeed (or sometimes fail), and they must avoid any opportunity to influence results.

12. *Patient specimens as ordinarily analyzed are the only basis for evaluating accuracy.* Although lyophilized preserved specimens are adequate for precision studies, they may yield significant bias from true values because they have been altered during processing. Such bias may be instrument-dependent or method-dependent. For example, we found the results using reconstituted materials were consistently higher with a narrow band-pass spectrophotometer than with a broad band-pass instrument, yet there was no difference when patient samples were analyzed.

13. Certain methods cannot be investigated by any of the techniques described above because the claims are clinical in nature. For example, pregnancy tests can only be validated by comparing the patients' clinical status with the test results. This is relatively easy because the outcome is obvious within nine months. On the other hand, suppose a test is alleged to detect early cancer. When we find a positive test we then proceed with a clinical investigation. How comprehensive must it be to prove that no cancer is present? For how long must we follow the patient? The difficulties are self-evident; the problem is not statistical but biological.

Outliers

In almost any series of analyses there are one or more obvious outliers, values which appear widely discordant from the others. The decision that such values can be eliminated is difficult. If there is collateral data to support the idea that a gross blunder was made, such as remembering that a wrong pipette was used, it is permissible to eliminate the value. If there are more than 3 obvious outliers in 40 patient comparisons, this alone should disqualify the test method because large random errors are medically very dangerous. If there are 3 or less outliers, arbitrary decisions must be made as to their importance; the outlier could result from an error in the reference method rather than the test method. Generally the arbitrary elimination of a single outlier can be done without much harm, but beyond that it is wise to include all the values obtained.

Evaluating the Results

We have now determined, as comprehensively as necessary and reasonable, the performance of the method we are testing, usually in parallel with a reference method. We are in an excellent position to decide whether it is suitable for our use. Several alternatives present themselves.

1. The test method is *as* accurate and precise as the reference method. We then can base our decision on other factors of convenience, economy, and so on.
2. The test method is significantly *more* accurate or precise than the reference method. If these factors are medically useful we should adopt the test method unless there are other significant drawbacks.
3. The test method is significantly *less* accurate or precise than the reference method. If the degree of inaccuracy is medically important we would not adopt the test method.

Statistical techniques as described will enable a decision to be made with full knowledge of many aspects of method performance. However, no statistical analysis will make an automatic value judgment about adoption of a method; to do this the laboratory director must consider all the other performance factors as well.

References

1. Barnett, R. N. A scheme for the comparison of quantitative methods. *Am. J. Clin. Pathol.* 43:562–569, 1965.
2. Barnett, R. N., and Cash, A. D. Performance of "kits" used for clinical chemical analysis of glucose. *Am. J. Clin. Pathol.* 52:457–465, 1969.
3. Barnett, R. N., Cash, A. D., and Junghans, S. P. Performance of "kits" used for clinical chemical analysis of cholesterol. *N. Engl. J. Med.* 279:974–979, 1968.
4. Barnett, R. N., Ewing, N. S., and Skodon, S. B. Performance of "kits" used for clinical chemical analysis of GOT (aspartate aminotransferase). *Clin. Biochem.* 9:78–84, 1976.
5. Barnett, R. N. and Youden, W. J. A revised scheme for the comparison of quantitative methods. *Am. J. Clin. Pathol.* 54:454–462, 1970.
6. Gilbert, R. K. *Survey Data Chemistry '74.* Skokie, Ill.: College of American Pathologists, 1975.

16 Simplified Laboratory Systems and Kits

Modern clinical laboratory testing is developing rapidly in two opposite directions. One is toward development of large, efficient, automated laboratories which do many tests very cheaply but require a large investment and specialized personnel; results may not be available locally or rapidly.

The other is toward production of simplified test systems that are relatively inexpensive, require a minimum of manipulation, produce results promptly, and can be operated by relatively unskilled persons. These test systems originally consisted of prepared reagents and instructions for their use. More recently they have often included photometers, disposable pipettes which may be self-filling, water-bath units to permit constant temperature heating, and reagent-filled disposable test tubes which also serve as cuvettes. They are marketed for small laboratories, such as physicians' offices, and for emergency or off-hours procedures in large laboratories.

We have been intimately concerned with testing these systems for the Product Evaluation Subcommittee of the College of American Pathologists since 1964, and for the Food and Drug Administration in 1966, 1967, and 1968. (The outline of the procedure followed is covered in Chapter 15.) Many pertinent facts became evident in the course of these studies.

1. There are satisfactory products on the market for most analyses commonly requested, if the term *satisfactory* is used to mean that accurate tests can be performed by careful and skilled personnel using the products.
2. There are unsatisfactory products on the market, and many others have been distributed but later abandoned. These unsatisfactory products are incapable of providing reliable results even in skilled hands. In our study of 12 cholesterol kits, 10 did not perform satisfactorily [2]; and of 17 glucose kits, 12 did not meet our arbitrary specifications based on comparisons with a reference method and on medical usefulness criteria [1].
3. None of the kits can be used properly unless the operator is skilled. The degree of skill required may not be great, but careful manipulation is always necessary, and the supervisor must understand the problems involved in order to recognize malfunctions.
4. Before the impact of FDA regulations began to be felt, there were frequent problems with poor operating instructions, lack of recommended quality control procedures, and inadequate supporting data for such performance claims as were provided. These problems have diminished markedly since 1971 and many products now provide excellent information.
5. For new products used to perform novel or difficult tests the supporting data are frequently inadequate or controversial and must be scrutinized very carefully.

Choice and Use of Kits

Chapter 15 discussed in detail the problems involved in choosing a method and how to solve them. The procedures entail considerable work in the laboratory, far more than most small installations care to undertake. Are there any reasonable alternatives?

Accept the advice of respected laboratories. This is what is done most often. The main weakness is that the procedure may not be carried out in exactly the same way; this can be checked by a relatively small number of comparison studies against a reference method or a reference laboratory.

Accept the statements of the manufacturer. If this is done, request comprehensive data of the type we have indicated—i.e., reproducibility, recovery, and patient comparison studies. Study the data for completeness and reasonableness. Unrealistically good performance should be suspect. For example, in one study we received, the analyst compared his own kit with a "reference method"—another kit! The results for individual samples always agreed within a few milligrams per 100 ml., which is far better agreement than can be achieved when repeated analyses are made by the same method, even the best. (The general performance levels which can be used as "state of the art" guides are listed in Chapter 19.) If the manufacturer has no data available or if it appears unsatisfactory, obviously his claims cannot be accepted.

Use products bearing the seal of the College of American Pathologists. For these products the manufacturer has submitted comprehensive claims which have been verified by an independent evaluator selected by the CAP. This means that the material is capable of performance as specified, at least in expert hands; it does not mean that any specific laboratory will use it as effectively. Again, at least a few comparison tests should be undertaken.

Test the system against samples of known content. This method is very satisfactory. Do not accept the labeled content of lyophilized commercial serum products as being gospel truth; usually this content provides a good approximation of the true value, but sometimes it is markedly different for certain methods.

Lot-to-Lot Variation

Even the most reliable manufacturer may market poor reagents occasionally. Some of the less-efficient producers do not have effective quality control from tube to tube and batch to batch. Sometimes this variability may be apparent on inspection, but more often it is difficult to detect. Use of proper internal quality control in the laboratory is the best safeguard against faulty reagents, whether they are supplied in kits or provided in some other fashion.

Generally, such products and systems made by ethical manufacturers can exert a favorable influence on laboratory practice by eliminating much tedious, repetitive reagent dispensing and by providing mass-production precision. This promising outlook, however, depends on the increasing application by industry of high-quality performance standards.

References

1. Barnett, R. N., and Cash, A. D. Performance of "kits" used for clinical chemical analysis of glucose. *Am. J. Clin. Pathol.* 52:457–465, 1969.
2. Barnett, R. N., Cash, A. D., and Junghans, S. P. Performance of "kits" used for clinical chemical analysis of cholesterol. *N. Engl. J. Med.* 279:974–979, 1968.

17 Computers in the Laboratory

The modern computer is a miraculous device well suited to clinical laboratory use. It can handle numbers, process them, and remember them incredibly accurately and rapidly. Because computers are so useful, many laboratories are already using them to a lesser or greater degree. Those statistical functions described in this book are ideally adapted to computers so we devote this brief chapter to a few relevant considerations.

A Few Terms

Computers may be of all sizes and competence; as various parts become miniaturized the smallest (*minicomputers*) can perform functions formerly requiring large (*main-frame*) instruments, and the performance lines are never sharply drawn.

To the extent that laboratory computers perform specific laboratory functions such as monitoring device output, calculating results and quality control, they should be *dedicated* to laboratory use. Attempts to perform such functions through an overall hospital computer CPU (central processing unit) have consistently failed. Among other defects many large computers are incapable of extensive mathematical calculations. Dedicated computers may actually be working parts of analytic devices, but are then not available for other uses. Some companies provide *turn-key* systems including the computers, programming (*software*), and necessary attachments for analytic devices; such systems are often inflexible and not adaptable to individual problems. The alternative is for the laboratory to secure its own equipment and programmer, to utilize available packaged programs, and to develop its own system. This is more difficult but gives a more personally tailored arrangement.

Computers may be *on-line*, picking signals directly from instruments, often via an interface, and calculating results promptly. Alternatively they may be *off-line* and accept input via a manual keyboard or via some form of tape.

A related device is the *programmable calculator*, not sharply delimited from the minicomputer, capable of being programmed to perform any of the calculations necessary for statistical analysis.

Before purchasing any type of laboratory computer it is well worth considering the subjects discussed below.

Systems Analysis

Systems analysis should precede purchase or installation of a computer; indeed, it may completely obviate the need for a computer. A simple example of this occurred in our histology laboratory. The problem was that all the surgical slides reached the desk of the surgical pathologist simultaneously at 2 P.M., so that he was relatively unoccupied before 2 P.M. and overwhelmed thereafter. The solution was not arrived at by hiring more technicians or buying more instruments, but rather by carefully studying the system itself. What was being done was that all the blocks were cut together, all the resultant sections were dried together, and then all were stained and delivered together. We changed this so that after each 20 blocks were cut, the sections were then dried and stained while the next 20 were being cut. In this way the surgical slides were sent out more or less continuously for reading from 11 A.M. until 2 P.M. This sort of batching to meet deadlines is equally applicable in Chemistry, where we now analyze the Intensive Care Unit electrolytes as soon as they are received rather than waiting to fill a 40-place tray.

Note that finding these problems and solving them are not computer functions. All too often a computer system, particularly a "turnkey" system pre-programmed for the "average" laboratory, does a marvelous job of solving all the nonexistent problems and ignoring the real ones. If your real problem is slowness in returning test results [1], you may merely need more frequent blood-drawing; a computer may not help at all. In fact, one system which we studied seemed calculated to slow the reporting; it stored test results in the main hospital computer, whence they were retrieved on a single daily report when the computer was not busy with more "urgent" tasks such as collecting financial data and billing.

Appropriate Use of the Laboratory Computer

Suppose that having now installed our own on-line computer after careful study, we are using it to provide better test procedures. The following are some specific procedures which are appropriate to our branch of statistics.

Randomizing quality-control samples. In using a 30- or 40-cup tray there is a human tendency to always place control samples first or at some other regular location. This defeats the original goal of assuring that all patient samples are analyzed properly. The computer work-sheet randomizes the location and specifies which cup is to receive which control.

Performing an "average of normals" calculation for each run. This is printed out at the end of the run as one of the quality-control parameters.

Identifying unacceptable runs. We worked out the following system, which could obviously be modified to meet other requirements. There are three parameters: a normal pool, an abnormal pool, and the average of normals. For each pool a result within $\pm 2 s$ limits is given 0 points, a result within $\pm 3 s$ limits but outside $\pm 2 s$ receives 1 point, and a result outside $\pm 3 s$ limits receives 2 points. An average of normals report outside $2 s$ is given 1 point. Any run having a score of 3 or more is considered unacceptable and all the test values are marked "rejected"; also, the words "reject run" appear on the printout.

Summarizing marginal and out-of-control data. Because we now acquire so much quality-control data on each run that it is difficult to monitor, we have a 4 P.M. printout which summarizes all marginal and out-of-control data for the day. This is used to review problems in order to discover if they are recurrent; it also serves as a permanent record for out-of-control values. A record of corrective action is requested and is entered on the form.

Reading curves closely. The computer input, working from the spindle of the ammeter indicator, reads more consistently than the human eye and avoids variations between different technicians reading the same points on a curve.

Drift correction. This is readily performed by a computer and is almost impossible without it.

Calculations. The computer can calculate final results from the data it acquires, avoiding the need for potentially erroneous manual calculations.

Identifying alarm values. These are starred and also printed out in a special section. The section has a space where the person who notifies the physician is asked to place his own name and the time of notification.

Checking values by their interrelationships. For instance, we presently set a goal for certain electrolytes such that the ion gap between sodium and the sum of chloride and bicarbonate should not stray beyond 12 ± 7 millimoles per liter. If the ion gap falls outside these limits the results are starred. Too many of these, if unexplained, point to systematic errors for one or more of the constituents and indicate that all the analyses require repetition. If a patient repeat gives the same results (outside the limits) the pathologist is notified and appropriate clinical investigation of the case is undertaken.

Entering daily quality-control pool values. These are collected in the computer and transmitted monthly to the regional pool headquarters.

Delta checks. In our next computer phase we will be able to compare a patient's values from one analysis to the next. Excessively large changes may indicate random laboratory errors or major physiologic disturbances which could require urgent treatment.

In summary, then, by using the computer as a statistical tool we can perform better analyses and monitor quality control more effectively. Because of its enormous storage capacity we can also use it for all sorts of calculations based on memory of past events. Please note that this discussion has not considered such valuable but nonstatistical functions as clerical functions, making printouts of patient reports, and recalling earlier test results for inspection.

References

1. Barnett, R. N., Bimmell, M., Peracca, M., and Rosemann, K. Time intervals between ordering and obtaining laboratory test results. *Lab. Med.* 7:18–21, 34, 1976.
2. Witte, D. L., Rodgers, J. L., and Barrett, D. A. II. The anion gap: Its use in quality control. *Clin. Chem.* 22:643–646, 1976.

III Application of Statistics in Patient Care

18 Application of Tests to Individual Patients

Accuracy of Single Results

Ideally when a physician receives a test result it should carry with it both the limits of experimental error and the limits of normal values. For example, it might read: "Fasting blood glucose—96 mg. per 100 ml. Standard deviation of determination—5 mg., so there is a 95 percent certainty that this value is between 86 and 106 mg. Normal limits for this patient's sex and age are 72 to 120 mg. per 100 ml."

Conveying both these parameters—precision and normal—on a single report sheet, however, becomes an impossible exercise in logistics. The data on precision, at one common level, at least, are available in the laboratory by perusal of the quality control pool confidence limits. Unfortunately, very few clinicians can make use of this knowledge; even if they are aware of its existence they do not have ready access to it. Probably every laboratory should publish its precision figures in the form of wallet cards or sheets to be posted in offices and on the wards. This information is essential for evaluation of repeated tests. For example, a patient is bleeding into the gastrointestinal tract and the hemoglobin drops from 12.0 to 11.0 gm. per 100 ml. Is this significant? If we know that s for hemoglobin is 0.17 gm., then a change of 1.0 gm. is over $5s$ and is unlikely to result from analytic error alone. It is possible that the patient's true hemoglobin was 11.5 and that the first reading was $3s$ high and the second $3s$ low. However, the probability of this is quite small, and one ordinarily assumes that a change greater than $3s$ between successive readings is meaningful. On the other hand, if s were 0.5 gm., then the change of $2s$ could easily result from analytic error.

Most clinicians achieve a subconscious understanding of these limits after dealing with the same laboratory for a while. It should be possible to formalize this and make it a conscious part of the decision process.

Influence of Extraneous Factors

One should not be so intrigued with the possibility of statistically evaluating day-to-day changes that he forgets all these tests are performed on materials from a living, varying body. Many test results are influenced vastly more by physiologic alterations than by analytic imprecision. For example, blood glucose levels are very labile, being markedly influenced not only by food but by emotion. Sieracki [4, 5] and his co-workers have demonstrated large rises in blood glucose due to emotion—even at the approach of a beautiful laboratory technician! Another common example is the fall of almost 1 gm. in blood hemoglobin when an ambulant patient lies down for a half-hour and extravascular fluid in his legs reenters the circulation. Fortunately, most body constituents are not so labile and good baseline conditions can be achieved. Any surprising change in the results of serial tests should be scrutinized carefully to find any factor in the disease process or the treatment which could have led to the change. Literally thousands of these factors exist.

Borderline Results

Using Venn diagrams to illustrate diagnostic tests, there are three possible patterns of test results (Fig. 18-1).

In type I, the ideal type from the viewpoint of laboratory diagnosis, there is no overlap. The healthy persons have low values; the diseased persons have high values. In Type II the test is useless. The values for healthy and diseased persons are identical. Type III is the usual type. Most healthy persons have low values, most diseased persons have high values, but there is a "gray" area at the intersection of the circles which includes high values from normal persons and low values from diseased persons. (Alternatively, healthy persons may have high values and diseased persons low ones.) The size of this gray zone may be very small or very large.

What are the chances that a value in the gray zone indicates disease? To calculate this we need to know the answers to two questions. First, what is the relative number of healthy and of sick persons in the population? Second, what is the mean and standard deviation for each group?

Example. Suppose we find a blood calcium value of 10.4 mg. per 100 ml. in a 40-year-old man. Patients with hypercalcemia represent about .17 percent of the population [1]. Normal calcium values are $\bar{x} = 9.2$, $s = 0.5$. Patients with hypercalcemia have an $\bar{x}$ of 11.5, $s = 0.5$. This is illustrated in Figure 18-2. 10.4 is 1.2 mg. higher, or $1.2/0.5 = 2.4s$ higher than the mean for normals. Looking in Appendix Table 6, Cumulative Normal Distribution, we find that the area above $\bar{x} + 2.4s$ represents only about .008 (by interpolation between .006 and .012) of

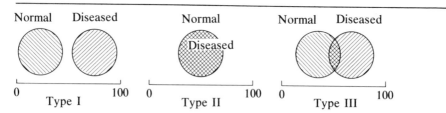

Figure 18-1
Venn diagrams indicating the three possible types of diagnostic test results. Type I, the ideal, shows no overlap of values for normal persons and those with disease. Type II is useless because there is complete overlap of normal and diseased persons. Type III is the usual situation in which some values are from normal persons, some from diseased persons, and some lie in an indeterminate region.

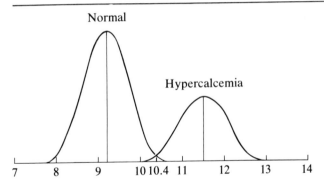

Figure 18-2
Interpretation of results (calcium, mg./100 ml.). Normal calcium levels are $\bar{x} = 9.2$ mg., $s = 0.5$. Hypercalcemic levels are $\bar{x} = 11.5$ mg., $s = 0.5$. The overlapping zone includes 10.4 mg., the value for the patient under study.

the total area, equivalent to .8 percent. Doing the same type of calculation for hypercalcemia, we find that 10.4 is 1.1 mg. or 2.2s lower than the mean, and the area below $\bar{x} - 2.2s$ represents about .014 of the total, equivalent to 1.4 percent. On this basis alone the odds favor hypercalcemia by 1.4/0.8 or 1.75 to 1. However, the normal population is 587 times as large as the sick population. The odds are then 587/1.75 or 335 to 1 that the value is from a normal person. Using these same values, and excluding analytic error, a true value of 9.5 has a 100 percent chance of representing a normal person, and one of 11.0 has a 100 percent chance of representing a hypercalcemic patient.

Similar calculations can be put in a Bayesian formula [3] or calculated as "predictive value" [6], but the principle is the same. The Bayesian formulas (after Hall [3]) are (1) the probability of the disease D_1 being present when a given value of S is observed, $p(D_1|S)$, and (2) the probability of the observation S arising in a group without the disease, $p(D_2|S)$.

Where $p(D_1)$ = incidence of disease D_1
$p(D_2)$ = incidence of nondisease D_2
S = a given variable
$p(S|D_1)$ = probability of S in disease D_1
$p(S|D_2)$ = probability of S in absence of disease D_1,

$$p\left(\frac{D_1}{S}\right) = \frac{p(D_1)p(S|D_1)}{p(D_1)p(S|D_1) + p(D_2)p(S|D_2)} \tag{1}$$

$$p\left(\frac{D_2}{S}\right) = \frac{p(D_2)p(S|D_2)}{p(D_2)p(S|D_2) + p(D_1)p(S|D_1)} \tag{2}$$

$p(S|D_1)$ and $p(S|D_2)$ are derived from probability tables. In the example we have used,

$$p\left(\frac{D_1}{S}\right) = \frac{(.0017 \times .014)}{(.0017 \times .014) + (.9983 \times .008)} = \frac{.0000238}{.0000238 + .0079864}$$

$$= \frac{238}{80,102} = .0029722$$

$$p\left(\frac{D_2}{S}\right) = \frac{(.9983 \times .008)}{(.9983 \times .008) + (.0017 \times .014)} = \frac{.0079864}{.0079864 + .0000238}$$

$$= \frac{79,864}{80,102} = .9970287$$

The odds then are 9,970,287/29,722 or 335 to 1 that the value comes from a normal person; this is the same result we obtained by using the normal curves.

Galen and Gambino [2] have expanded the concept of predictive value into a small monograph in which they give examples derived from different laboratory tests. The terms *sensitivity*,* meaning ability to detect an abnormal state (true positives) by a particular test and *specificity*, meaning ability to obtain normal results in nondiseased populations (true negatives), are used extensively. In the Bayesian formulas given above, sensitivity is portrayed by $p(S|D_1)$, and specificity by $1 - p(S|D_2)$. The authors also provided a large number of tables relating predictive value to sensitivity and specificity for various disease prevalences. One problem with these tables is that prevalence is rarely known with any accuracy, but the overall approach is useful.

We must not forget that a single determination has an intrinsic imprecision. In our example we assumed that the determined value is the true value, but this could be incorrect, as we described earlier. When any borderline value is encountered the best procedure is to repeat it, particularly if an important action may follow from knowledge of the result.

At this point we enter the realm of medical usefulness and ask What do we propose to do with the result? In the example just given the existence of unexplained hypercalcemia calls for thorough investigation. If no other cause is identified we assume that the patient has a parathyroid lesion requiring surgery; the surgery is difficult and may be very extensive. It is therefore essential that the existence of hypercalcemia be proven beyond reasonable doubt, preferably by repeated analyses at intervals of at least a few days.

Suppose we chose a different example, namely a serum uric acid of 7.5 mg. per 100 ml. in a 45-year-old man; normal 95 percent limits are 3.0 to 6.7 mg. In an asymptomatic patient, given our present state of knowledge, there seems no reason to do anything therapeutically with either diet or drugs; there is no need

---

*This use of the term *sensitivity* must be clearly distinguished from the chemical usage, meaning the lowest concentration at which an analyte can be detected.

for repeating the test. To expand this example, suppose the uric acid were 9.0 mg. We believe that at this level the patient has a 50 percent chance of developing clinical gout in the near future. We would now be justified in repeating the test on several occasions, and if we substantiated the first report we would proceed with prophylactic medication.

To summarize this discussion, statistical processes can be employed very fruitfully in considering the significance of single normal, borderline, or abnormal values, but the extent to which investigation is pursued is determined primarily by clinical considerations.

References

1. Boonstra, E. E., and Jackson, E. E. The clinical value of routine serum calcium analyses. *Ann. Intern. Med.* 57:963–969, 1962.
2. Galen, R. S., and Gambino, S. R. *Beyond Normality: The Predictive Value and Efficiency of Medical Diagnoses.* New York: Wiley, 1975.
3. Hall, G. H. Laboratory data and diagnosis. *Lancet* 1:531, 1969.
4. Sieracki, J. C., Sabek, G. A., Danowski, T. S., Spicker, J., Walsh, J. A., and Sadlowe, C. S. Individual Health Research Program. Pilot Phase: Continuous Analysis of Multiple Blood Parameters. II. In Vivo Studies on Human Subjects. Scientific paper 106 presented at ASCP-CAP meeting, Miami Beach, Fla., Oct. 17, 1968.
5. Sieracki, J. C., Sabek, G. A., Danowski, T. S., and Walsh, J. A. Individual Health Research Program. Pilot Phase: Continuous Analysis of Multiple Blood Parameters. III. Intraindividual Correlations and Comparison of Dynamic vs. Static (Discrete) Measurements. Scientific paper 107 presented at ASCP-CAP meeting, Miami Beach, Fla., Oct. 17, 1968.
6. Vecchio, T. J. Predictive value of a single diagnostic test in unselected populations. *N. Engl. J. Med.* 274:1171–1173, 1966.

19 Medical Usefulness and Choice of Tests

One cannot dissociate the choice of test procedures from the use to which the test results will be put. The concepts in this chapter were derived by the Subcommittee on Criteria of Medical Usefulness of the College of American Pathologists [1] in evaluating this problem, with particular application to the effects of government-required proficiency surveys.

The term *decision level* refers to levels at which medical decisions are made concerning *diagnosis or treatment*. They are therefore of more critical importance than are some other levels.

The nine guidelines which were laid down by the Subcommittee and the pertinent discussion follow.*

A. *Desirable limits for accuracy and precision must be defined individually for each type of analysis performed.*

   Comment: It would be most convenient if a single set of limits could be applied to every type of analysis. This is impossible. Some clinical laboratory analyses are reported quantitatively, and others as positive or negative; others require value judgments as to exact identification of lesions, cells, or organisms.

   Even within the primarily quantitative disciplines such as clinical chemistry and hematology, significant limits differ for different substances.

   1. Some differences are technical in nature, reflecting the much greater precision of certain analytic technics. The thinking of attending physicians over the years reflects their observation of this fact; they draw conclusions from small changes in values for some tests and not for others. When better methods are introduced, clinicians utilize the greater precision by appropriate changes in their interpretation of results.
   2. Other differences are physiologic. For calcium, a substance which is under close homeostatic control, a very precise technic is most desirable. For glucose, a substance whose blood level varies widely depending on ingestion of food, emotion, time of day, and other factors, such great precision of analysis is not helpful in the interpretation of test results.

B. *Desirable limits for accuracy and precision must be defined at each level of medical significance. Maximal accuracy and precision are necessary at decision levels.*

   Comment: For example, the bilirubin determination decision levels are at about 1.2 mg. per 100 ml., separating normal from hyperbilirubinemic individuals, and at about 20.0 mg. per 100 ml., the critical level for embarking on exchange transfusion of erythroblastotic infants. At these levels physicians require the greatest accuracy because vital decisions depend on the results. On the other hand, at such intermediate levels as 9.0 mg. per 100 ml. no change in diagnosis or treatment would follow a relatively large change in the reported result. Another example is in glucose determination. A 2-hour postprandial plasma glucose of 120 mg. per 100 ml. is accepted as normal; a level of 130 mg. per 100 ml. leads to further consideration of possible diabetes, so that 120 mg. represent a decision level. A much larger difference

*From Barnett [1] (Reproduced with permission from the *American Journal of Clinical Pathology*, Volume 50, pp. 671–676; 1968).

between 200 mg. per 100 ml. and 250 mg. per 100 ml. would alter neither diagnosis nor treatment.

C. *Accuracy and precision of a degree greater than is useful clinically should not be required if extra time or expense is thereby made necessary.*

   Comment: Erythrocyte counts done in a single chamber are not accurate enough to be clinically useful. If four chambers are counted and the values averaged, a useful but expensive result is achieved. As technology improved, automatic counting devices appeared and the results became both cheap and clinically useful. Another example is identification of *Salmonella*. Knowledge that a stool culture contains a *Salmonella* grouped by group serum and biochemical reactions is medically vital information. Further complete identification is not necessary for patient care, despite the epidemiologic information provided; it is also prohibitively expensive in hospital practice. Antigen analysis therefore should not be obligatory for ordinary medical care facilities.

D. *Desirable accuracy should be such that the method will create no substantial divergence from generally accepted values for normal and disease states.*

   Comment: For many nonenzyme constituents of body fluids physicians have learned normal ranges. It is not proper to adopt a new method yielding different ranges unless there are substantial advantages in accuracy, precision, ease, rapidity of performance, or freedom from [outliers]. If a truly advantageous method is developed and introduced a thorough explanation must be made to clinicians. This was done, for example, when "true" glucose methods replaced Folin-Wu technics. Pressure to change to new technics yielding different normals should not be applied unless medical benefits are clearly promoted thereby.

E. *Desirable precision should be such that errors induced by the measurement process do not significantly widen the range of values for the normal population.*

   Comment: This objective is achieved by methods whose standard deviation does not exceed one-twelfth to one-twentieth of the normal population range defined as including 95% of normal persons. The "normal" range is a composite of true differences between individuals and of differences introduced by the technical methods. If the standard deviation of the method is one-twelfth of the population range it will cause the apparent range to be 5.4% larger than the true range; if it is one-twentieth of the population range it will cause an enlargement of 2.0%. This particular criterion is less reliable than the others noted because our present knowledge of normal ranges is inadequate and uncertain. If the normal range were compiled for a group uniform as to sex, age, ethnic group, and geographic location, it would be narrower than the usual range for all adults. Goals for precision in this category would therefore differ, depending on the population chosen.

F. *Ability to distinguish normal from abnormal values is often more important than the determination of absolute values.*

   Comment: For some substances in body fluids there are many analytic methods yielding widely disparate numerical results. Enzyme analyses fall into this category. Even laboratories allegedly using identical methods rarely achieve identical results, yet most of them distinguish adequately between normal and abnormal values—this is the information which the attending physician needs.

G. *An approximate result available promptly may be much more useful than an exact result reported after a long delay.*

Comment: Two examples will illustrate this point clearly.

1. In an unconscious diabetic patient an immediate report that the blood glucose is very low is an invaluable guide to prompt treatment and may be lifesaving. Conversely, a precise report that the glucose level is 20.3 mg. per 100 ml. is useless if it is not available until 24 hr. later, when the patient is dead.
2. A Gram stain of purulent spinal fluid correctly and immediately reported as demonstrating Gram-positive lanceolate diplococci is vital information for initiating treatment. If the full report of *Diplococcus pneumoniae* Type 18 is delayed for 2 days it is useless.

H. *An approximate result available locally under usual laboratory conditions may be more useful medically than a more accurate value available only at a distant center.*

Comment: Here the medical use to which the result is to be put is crucial. Again blood glucose is an example; a crude method which can be performed with locally available personnel and equipment is necessary to save lives. On the other hand, a crude protein-bound iodine method would never be justified because delay in reporting of mailed-out specimens will not harm the patient.

I. *A less precise analytic technic free of large error may be preferable to a more precise method subject to [erratic performance].*

This aspect of analytic technics has not received adequate attention. It is particularly important for tests in which a sudden large shift of values or a single abnormal result may lead to immediate therapeutic or diagnostic decisions. Some technical factors which lead to [erratic performance] are: complex or difficult instrument manipulations, too many steps in the procedure, and intricate calculations of results.

Specific Limits for Medical Significance

[Table 19-1] is a synthesis of opinions by clinicians and laboratory specialists. It lists 16 commonly tested blood constituents (Column 1) at 23 decision levels (Column 2). Column 3 gives the appropriate standard deviation at the corresponding decision level and represents what would be clinically expected for ordinary use, that is, that 95% of analytic values would be within $\pm 2s$ of the true value. Column 4 is the coefficient of variation calculated from Columns 2 and 3. Column 5 is a list of "low" values below which accuracy is unnecessary; a report that the concentration is this value or lower is adequate for medical purposes.

Intralaboratory and Interlaboratory Evaluation

Precision within a single laboratory is inevitably superior to that between laboratories, no matter how excellent their performance, because interlaboratory differences result from systematic bias. For example, let us assume that five competent laboratories analyze a sample of serum for glucose, each with a day-to-day precision of 2 mg. for 1 s. However, the mean values are 90, 94, 98, 102, and 106 mg./100 ml., respectively. A physician who used any one of these laboratories routinely would be able to use the normal and abnormal results readily. However, in a survey, if the mean value were 98, and only values of 94 and 102 were thereby accepted as satisfactory by using the precision of a single laboratory, 60% of the values for these five laboratories would be outside the 2s range of the mean. It is necessary, therefore, to use a system based on results of all participants to incorporate both interlaboratory and intralaboratory variability into proficiency evaluation.

Table 19-1
Medical Significance Values

Component	Decision Level*	s at Same Level†	Calculated CV (%)	Low Level*
Hemoglobin	10.5 gm.	0.5	4.76	5 gm.
Hematocrit	32%	1.0	3.12	10%
Glucose	50 mg.	5.0	10.00	20 mg.
Glucose	100 mg.	5.0	5.00	
Glucose	120 mg.	5.0	4.17	
Blood urea nitrogen	27 mg.	2.0	7.41	4 mg.
Uric acid	6.0 mg.	0.5	8.33	4 mg.
Total protein	7.0 gm.	0.3	4.28	2 gm.
Albumin	3.5 gm.	0.25	7.14	1.5 gm.
Globulin	3.5 gm.	0.25	7.14	1.5 gm.
Cholesterol	250 mg.	20.0	8.00	80 mg.
Bilirubin	1.0 mg.	0.2	20.00	0.4 mg.
Bilirubin	20.0 mg.	1.5	7.50	
Calcium	11.0 mg.	0.25	2.27	5.0 mg.
Phosphorus	4.5 mg.	0.25	5.56	1.5 mg.
Sodium	130 mEq./l.	2.0	1.54	100 mEq./l.
Sodium	150 mEq./l.	2.0	1.33	
Potassium	3 mEq./l.	0.25	8.33	1.5 mEq./l.
Potassium	6 mEq./l.	0.25	4.17	
Chloride	90 mEq./l.	2.0	2.22	50 mEq./l.
Chloride	110 mEq./l.	2.0	1.82	
CO_2	20 mEq./l.	1.0	5.00	8 mEq./l.
CO_2	30 mEq./l.	1.0	3.33	

*All values per 100 ml. unless indicated.
†Same units as corresponding decision level.
Source: Barnett [1] (Reproduced with permission from the *American Journal of Clinical Pathology,* Volume 50, pp. 671–676, 1968).

Utilization of Specific Limits in Medical Practice

It is best if the practicing physician knows the normal values and precision for the clinical laboratory which he uses most often. If he does not have these data, or is presented with values from another laboratory, he can use [Table 19-2] by observing the following simple rules.

Table 19-2
Comparison of 1967 CV Limits for Most Precise Method with
"Medically Significant CV"

1 Component and Level*	2 Medically Significant CV (%)	3 State of the Art CV (%)	4 Percent of Participant Values Excluded 3 vs. 2
Hemoglobin, 10.5 gm.	4.8	3.5	0
Glucose, 100 mg.	5.0	5.3	1.4
Glucose, 120 mg.	4.2	5.2	6.1
Blood urea nitrogen, 27 mg.	7.4	8.3	3.0
Uric acid, 6.0 mg.	8.3	5.8	0
Total protein, 7.0 gm.	4.3	3.9	0
Albumin, 3.5 gm.	7.1	8.8	6.2
Globulin, 3.5 gm.	7.1	8.8	6.2
Cholesterol, 250 mg.	8.0	9.1	3.3
Bilirubin, 1.0 mg.	20.0	23.3	4.0
Bilirubin, 20.0 mg.	7.5	12.8	19.7
Calcium, 11.0 mg.	2.3	2.8	5.7
Phosphorus, 4.5 mg.	5.6	8.4	13.7
Sodium, 130 mEq./l.	1.5	1.8	4.9
Sodium, 150 mEq./l.	1.3	2.0	14.8
Potassium, 3 mEq./l.	8.3	3.7	0
Potassium, 6 mEq./l.	4.2	3.3	0
Chloride, 90 mEq./l.	2.2	2.1	0
Chloride, 110 mEq./l.	1.8	2.1	4.2

*All values per 100 ml. unless indicated.
Note: For CAP proficiency surveys, values outside ±2 CV calculated from Column 3 are considered to be not acceptable, thus excluding 4.55% of all results. If Column 2 values were to be used to evaluate survey performance, an additional percentage of participant values as indicated in Column 4 would be considered not acceptable.
Source: Barnett [1] (Reproduced with permission from the *American Journal of Clinical Pathology*, Volume 50, pp. 671–676, 1968).

1. Find the component and the nearest level in Column 1.
2. Take the corresponding CV in Column 3 and double it. The correct value for any result will almost [always] lie within plus or minus the percentage just calculated. (Example: A uric acid is reported as 7.0 mg./100 ml. We take the 5.8% in Column 3; double it to get 11.6; the 7.0 mg. figure is almost certainly between $7 \times 0.116 = 0.81$ above or below 7.0; i.e., between 6.19 and 7.81.)
3. For substances whose Column 4 value is 0% or near it, the laboratory accuracy is adequate for your use. If the Column 4 value is high and the decision vital, repeat the analysis several times. For example, if hyperparathyroidism is suspected and a calcium level of 10.8 is found, at least two repeat samples should be examined before the disease is considered to be excluded or demonstrated as far as the calcium level is concerned.

These guidelines permit alteration as the state of the art improves. They should not be used as an excuse for use of poor procedures if better ones are available. For most tests which are vital to medical care on an emergency basis, excellent reagent sets are presently produced that contain prepackaged reagents in convenient form.

Reference

1. Barnett, R. N. Medical significance of laboratory results. *Am. J. Clin. Pathol.* 50:671–676, 1968.

20 Multiphasic Screening by Laboratory Tests

There is a complex reciprocal relationship between technologic capability and medical practice. The need for laboratory diagnostic tests led industry to develop remarkable machinery for performing these tests; in turn the capability of the automated, computerized laboratory to turn out enormous quantities of reasonably accurate results at low cost has encouraged physicians and public health authorities to perform "mass testing." Subjects for these procedures may be whole populations, healthy persons being examined in physicians' offices, or hospital patients who are tested for abnormalities not necessarily related to their major illness. The concept of screening hospital patients is an old one; traditionally a complete blood count and urinalysis have been required as a routine admission procedure. With the new methodology this can be expanded to encompass a wide variety of procedures, most biochemical. The possibilities of this technic as an investigative tool are enormous and are being widely explored. Before it is accepted for routine use [1], many questions need be answered. They include the following: (1) What tests shall we do? (2) Under what conditions shall we do them? (3) What shall we do with the results?

Choice of Tests

Choice of tests should be determined by demonstrated medical usefulness rather than by instrument capability. Although this seems self-evident it is widely disregarded. The following criteria should be utilized:

The test must usually yield abnormal results in the presence of one or more specific diseases or disease conditions generally.

There should be few or no abnormal results in persons free of disease or a definite predisposition to disease. Assume for example that a test yields 2 percent false positives, that the true incidence of the disease is 1 percent of the population, and that false negatives do not occur. If we test 1,000 persons we will encounter 10 with disease who will react positively, and 2 percent of 990 or 20 false positives, for a total of 30 positives. The 20 false reactors must undergo further studies which will be a nuisance, often expensive, and which may be psychologically and physically distressing or even actually hazardous.

The condition associated with abnormal results must be reasonably common. Note in the example just given that there were 10 true positives for 20 false positives. Suppose the true disease incidence had been 0.1 percent instead of 1 percent. We would have then detected 21 positives, of which only 1 would have been a true positive. The definition of *reasonably common*, then, rests both on statistical grounds determined by the incidence of false reactions and on economic grounds determined by the expense of finding each verified case.

The conditions associated with abnormal results must be significant to health. Many physical and chemical differences between individuals are interesting but unimportant.

The conditions associated with abnormal results must be reasonably amenable to treatment or prevention. This must be interpreted broadly; diseases which are incurable today may be successfully treated next year. Sometimes early diagnosis of incurable disease permits physicians to give useful advice about job and estate planning. The hazard of producing national neuroses in an already neurotic society must be considered seriously, however; the benefits of presymptomatic detection should be balanced against this hazard.

In general then the choice of tests is useful to the degree that the tests are specific and the conditions to be identified are common, important to health, and treatable.

Conditions of Sampling and Performance

The conditions of sampling must be clearly specified. If glucose or BUN is tested postprandially, the expected values will be different from fasting values. For postprandial glucose particularly, choice of challenge dose material and time after the dose are critical.

The accuracy and precision of the method chosen must be specified. Screening tests in which minor differences from normal are sought may require better methods than those for patient care in which overt disease often produces major deviations from the normal.

Use of the Results

Definition of Normal Limits

Normal limits must be clearly defined, as discussed elsewhere. They must be defined to correspond to the same conditions of sampling and performance which are applied to the individuals tested. Assuming that $\pm 2s$ limits are used to define the normal range, then for each test 4.55 percent of the values are considered abnormal. If multiple tests are used, we can calculate as follows the chances that any one person will demonstrate all normal values:

For one test we exclude 4.55 percent, leaving 95.45 percent. For a second test we exclude 4.55 percent of the remaining 95.45 percent or 4.343 percent, leaving 94.45 percent minus 4.343 percent or 91.107 percent normal for the two tests, and we continue in this manner. Table 20-1 specifies the percentages of the original population which would be normal for the given number of tests if the tests were all independent variables. If there were any relationship between the different tests, so that a high value for test A often accompanied a high value for test B, then the proportion of persons who were normal for all tests would be higher than that tabulated.

Table 20-1
Percentage of Persons Expected To Be Normal for a Number of Tests,
Each Using $\bar{x} \pm 2s$ Normal Range

Number of Different Tests	Persons Expected To Be Normal for All Tests Undertaken (%)
1	95.45
2	91.11
3	86.96
4	83.00
5	79.23
6	75.62
7	72.18
8	68.90
9	65.76
10	62.77
11	59.91
12	57.19

Getting the Physician's Attention

If a large amount of data reaches the busy practitioner's desk he may easily overlook the abnormal values, thus defeating the whole purpose of screening. Williamson et al. [5] found that this actually occurs. In a group of hospital patients, two-thirds of the abnormal results for blood glucose, routine urinalysis, and hemoglobin determination elicited no physician response.

Some means of dramatizing abnormal values is needed. The methods which have been tried include graphic charts of different sorts, asterisks or different-colored ink for abnormals, and use of units reported in terms of normal range rather than exact chemical levels [3]. This problem should be readily soluble by modern technology.

Follow-up of Abnormal Values

Following up abnormal values is the most difficult and crucial task. If it is not carried out assiduously the entire program is one of meaningless data collection. Table 20-2 shows what actually happened when Dr. Young [6] reported the results of a large number of tests to a group of clinicians in Toronto. This rather discouraging picture indicates that only 3 percent of the patients received a new diagnosis as a result of the many "unsolicited" tests performed. One can only hope that screening laboratory tests under different circumstances will be followed up more successfully and yield more useful information.

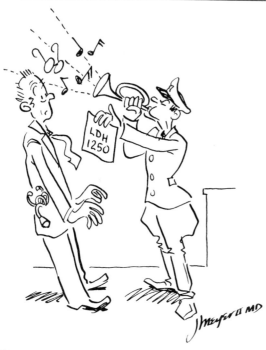

GETTING THE PHYSICIAN'S ATTENTION

Table 20-2
Results of Performing Unsolicited Tests on 1,010 Patients*

Original number of patients	1,010
A. No abnormalities	228
B. Abnormalities expected	140
C. Physician rejected at least one item as error, others normal	182
D. Abnormalities unexpected, required decision as to further procedures	430
1. Not followed up	253
2. Followed up	177
a. Pending at time of study	27
b. Patient did not return	55
c. Investigated further	95
(1) Disease identified	27
3. Chart reviewed, led to further investigation not related to abnormal laboratory value	30

*Data from Young, Drake, and Weir [6].

Stability of Values in Individual Persons

There is some dispute about the stability of values in individuals. The usual belief is that levels in healthy individuals remain reasonably constant. Glassy and Blumenfeld [2] followed 12 persons at weekly intervals for about three years and demonstrated considerable stability for the following constituents: glucose, BUN, uric acid, cholesterol, GOT, alkaline phosphatase, total protein, albumin, globulin, calcium, magnesium, protein electrophoresis, leukocytes, erythrocytes, hemoglobin, hematocrit, and leukocyte differential count. However, there are known to be substantial changes in glucose, uric acid, and cholesterol depending on stress, emotion, and physical activity, all difficult to control in mass screening. Mefferd and Pokorny [4] in a minority opinion found that variation in a single individual was as great as that in a group of individuals for many biochemical constituents of the body. If this is true then effective screening would have to be repeated frequently to overcome these fluctuations from time to time.

To summarize, mass screening is a potentially useful technique which will find its real role after many practical problems are solved.

References

1. Barnett, R. N., Civin, W. H., and Schoen, I. Multiphasic screening by laboratory tests—an overview of the problem. *Am. J. Clin. Pathol.* 54:483–492, 1970.
2. Glassy, F. J., and Blumenfeld, C. M. Individual normal laboratory values: Preliminary observations. *Calif. Med.* 108:172–178, 1968.
3. Hoffman, R. G., and Waid, M. E. A new scale of normal values for physicians. *G. P.* 30:112–121, 1964.
4. Mefferd, R. B., and Pokorny, A. D. Individual variability reexamined with standard clinical measures. *Am. J. Clin. Pathol.* 48:325–331, 1967.
5. Williamson, J. W., Alexander, M., and Miller, G. E. Continuing education and patient care research: Physician response to screening test results. *J.A.M.A.* 201:118–122, 1967.
6. Young, D. M., Drake, N., and Weir, R. J. The advent of chemical screening techniques. *Can. Med. Assoc. J.* 98:868–870, 1968.

IV Statistics for Manufacturers

21 Statistics for Manufacturers

Makers of laboratory instruments, equipment, and reagents use statistics constantly in three contexts: product development, quality control, and assuring conformance to governmental or other specifications.

Product Development and Claims Verification

The approaches discussed in Chapters 15 and 16 are aimed at the user of laboratory supplies but are equally pertinent to the manufacturer. New products which are similar to ones already described should be tested for precision, bias compared to accepted methods, recovery of added pure analyte, known or suspected interferences, and range of linearity. Products that quantify analytes for which there is no satisfactory accepted method must be tested primarily for their ability to detect correct amounts of known analyte in pure solutions or of known analyte added to base materials (recovery experiments).

In developing a new product for a common analyte, it is important to be familiar with the current performance of existing products. Such information—by analyte, by method, and by specific product—is published quarterly in the CAP Survey Reports to Participants and annually in CAP Survey Data. These data include precision and bias information.

One step which is absolutely essential but frequently neglected is the field trial—in which a new commercial product is evaluated in a laboratory other than the one where the method was developed. Such a field test may be conducted in a separate laboratory at the manufacturing plant, but it is more reliable when an entirely different facility is selected, preferably one appropriate for the contemplated general use of the product. Only in this fashion can one detect poor instructions for test procedures, deterioration in the field, problems with different spectrophotometers, and the myriad variables which characterize clinical laboratories.

One such outside testing agency is the Product Evaluation Committee of the College of American Pathologists.* This continuing committee provides to manufacturers a private source which will evaluate products submitted to it, verify the claims made, and permit promotional use of the verification. The committee has conducted testing of various products since 1964 and has evolved a reliable approach described below.

1. The manufacturer provides claims for operational and performance characteristics based on actual trial. The evaluator then repeats the experiments and either verifies or fails to verify the claims.

*College of American Pathologists Product Evaluation Program, College of American Pathologists, 7400 N. Skokie Blvd., Skokie, Ill. 60076.

2. The claims are discussed in advance by the manufacturer and the evaluator, because these claims must be medically pertinent and scientifically valid. There must be agreement on such details as the choice of reference method; the levels at which testing is carried out; and the numbers, types, and numerical distribution of patient samples. This conference provides a forum for agreement on how specific products are to be used in clinical situations; this use varies considerably for different types of products.

Few manufacturers evolve suitable claims in their first experience with this system; indeed, on occasion the Committee has considered claims which were meaningless even if verifiable. Claims which conform to the principles described in Chapter 15 are usually suitable. *Operational claims*—such as speed and simplicity of test performance and instrument characteristics—are easily verified and appeal to marketing personnel; they are not usually germane to the performance claims but often outweigh them in advertising copy. It is the *performance claims* which are vital in establishing the validity of the technique, and it is these which will ultimately be scrutinized by outside agencies such as the federal government. We will consider the present Food and Drug Administration (FDA) approach later in this chapter.

If the consulting laboratory fails to verify the claims, a reason for the discrepancy should be found. Often there was a procedural difference because the manufacturer's analysts used a technique whose details were quite obvious to them but which were not described clearly enough in the instructions. Sometimes the original testing was done on a pilot batch of reagents which were not reproduced correctly in the production run. Occasionally the original analysts were so anxious to please their employer that they used "within-run" rather than "between-run" values, or improved their results in some other fashion. Sometimes the Product Evaluation Laboratory failed to carry out analyses properly. Whatever the reason, it must be found and corrected, and the evaluation must be repeated, lest there be need for "recalls" similar to those frequently issued for automobiles! If the evaluating laboratory finds, for example, that the CV is 5 percent rather than the 2 percent originally claimed, the claim can be corrected to read 5 percent, which is then verifiable.

Quality Control

Quality control in the manufacturing process is discussed extensively in other works, so we will treat it lightly here. Obviously, each element or ingredient of the instrument or reagent must be carefully controlled within specified limits if the system is to work properly. Some specifications must be very rigid, others are less demanding, and only experiment will suffice to set appropriate limits. The final proof is the end result, i.e., How good are the final analytic results?

Once it is determined that certain limits are adequate—for example, that a reagent pH of 6 to 7 units is needed, then a system for assuring maintenance of this pH must be established and followed [1, 2]. In deciding which factors need be monitored, a Latin Square design as described by Youden can be employed economically to discover which elements are critical and which are not (see Chapter 7, Multiple Variables, pp. 68–72). Batch testing may require considerable ingenuity, but the statistical principles of quality control for manufacturers are no different than those described for laboratory procedures (Chapter 10).

Specifications and Conformance to Them

There is no difference in the general plan for verifying performance, whether this verification be done to assure compliance with a preset standard (as in the proposed FDA system for Product Class Standards) or to assure compliance with a manufacturer's claim submitted to the CAP Product Evaluation Program. In essence there are two steps:

1. The manufacturer provides data on the performance of his product for certain parameters such as accuracy, precision, and interference by certain substances.
2. The outside agency decides whether the data submitted verify the performance claimed or required. The agency may also perform its own analyses to validate the data.

The Development and Meaning of Claims

We have illustrated in Chapter 15 the statistics necessary to develop claims for accuracy by comparison to a reference method, by recovery experiments, and by determination of reproducibility. Chapter 15 also indicated the precautions to be followed in assuring that the experiments themselves were properly done so that statistical analysis would be valid. Assuming that these experiments have been carried out properly, we have then proceeded to establish such claims as the following:

1. The difference between the test method results and the XYZ reference method results indicate a bias of 2 mg. at a mean level of 100 mg., the test method results being higher.
2. The day-to-day precision of the test method is 5 percent CV at the 50 mg. level, 4 percent CV at the 100 mg. level, and 3 percent CV at the 150 mg. level.

Note that these claims give specific levels and specific reference methods so that an evaluator could reproduce the experiments. However, the information still lacks one dimension necessary to permit comparison with standards or with a similar experiment carried out independently. Specifically, what are the confidence limits for each of these claims? And what are the chances that an independent experiment would validate them?

Taking the second question first, consider as an example the 4 percent CV found at the 100 mg. level. Suppose the standard demanded a maximum 5 percent CV as a performance requirement. Is it possible that on 100 repetitions of the study the true CV of the test would be found to exceed 5 percent? What the foregoing claim data provided is called "parameter estimation"; what the question asks for is the result of something called "hypothesis testing" that requires a much more extensive set of studies. For example, a model proposed by an FDA statistician could require from 360 to 1,440 individual analyses to determine conformance, whereas our original study outlined in Chapter 15 needed only 220 individual analyses. In "hypothesis testing" one first decides the element of risk to be taken. The decision might be that if 5 percent CV were the maximum permitted, the hypothesis testing would falsely demonstrate nonconformance in only 5 percent of the experiments if the true value were 4 percent CV, and would demonstrate conformance in only 5 percent of the experiments if the true CV were 6 percent. This can be illustrated by the operating characteristics curves shown in Figure 21-1.

Assume that curve 1 is based on 10 df, curve 2 on 25 df, and curve 3 on 100 df. If we did 26 analyses (25 df) to compare to curve 2 values, and if we obtained a CV of 3 percent, there would only be a 2.5 percent chance of the analysis being rejected on subsequent testing if the acceptable value were 5 percent CV. However, if we performed only 11 analyses (10 df) and obtained a CV of 3

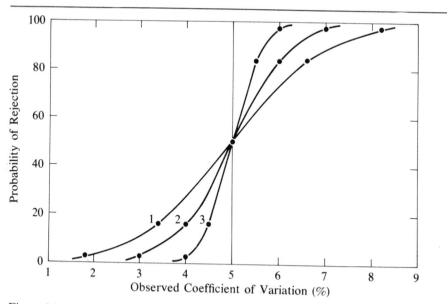

Figure 21-1

Family of operating characteristics curves in which acceptable CV is 5%. The probability of rejecting experimentally obtained CV's is indicated on the ordinate. Curve 1 is for 10 df, Curve 2 is for 25 df, and Curve 3 is for 100 df.

percent, there would be a 10 percent chance of subsequent rejection (curve 1); and if we performed 101 analyses (100 df) and found a CV of 3 percent, there would be essentially no chance of subsequent rejection (Curve 3). Therefore, the number of experiments needed to affirm the original hypothesis would be somewhere between 26 and 101.

But what are the confidence limits for the original claims? We can determine this from Appendix Table 7. This table gives upper and lower limits for various degrees of freedom and degrees of confidence.

Illustrative Problems

Acceptable Precision

Assume that the FDA sets a glucose product class standard of 4.0 mg. as acceptable for one standard deviation (between day) at the 100 mg. per dl. level. The manufacturer tested his product and obtained the results shown in Table 10-1 (p. 94). Would the 3.007 mg. value found be acceptable as meeting the 4.0 mg. criterion? We would like to be 95 percent confident that it was, so that if another batch of 20 replicates were tested there would not be more than a 5 percent chance of exceeding 4.0 mg.

We refer to Appendix Table 7 and find that at 19 df the upper limit for 95 percent confidence is 1.358 (this table lists 20 as the closest to the 19 desired, so use the number under 20 df). We therefore multiply this figure by 3.007 found by experiment and find the upper limit to be 4.08, which slightly exceeds 4.0. Therefore we cannot be certain that we have met the criterion at the 95 percent confidence level. Our next step, then, is to do more tests. We find that for 25 df the table factor becomes 1.308; this, when multiplied by 3.007, gives 3.93, a result which is less than 4.0. Therefore we perform 6 more analyses. If s has not increased we have established our desired degree of confidence with 26 analyses. If we wished to be 99 percent confident we would search the $A_{.99}$ column in Table 7 for a value close to 1.308; we would find that for 50 analyses the factor is 1.297. Thus if s remained the same for 50 analyses, we could then be 99 percent confident of meeting the requirement.

Acceptable Accuracy

Suppose the FDA permits a maximum bias of 12 mg. for glucose analysis products at the 120 mg. per dl. level when patient samples are analyzed by two methods, an approved reference method and a test method. Assume the manufacturer obtained the values given in Table 15-1 (p. 136), the "old method" being the reference method and the "new method" the test method. He found that for these 10 comparisons there was a bias of 9.6 mg. and that the standard deviation of the differences (s_d) was 5.10. The t test as calculated on page 135 yielded a result of 5.95, so there was a proven bias between the two methods.

The question, however, is not whether a bias exists, but whether the 9.6 mg.

bias is less than the 12 mg. permitted in the hypothetical example. We can calculate this by using the t test formula

$$t = \frac{\text{diff } \sqrt{n}}{s_d}$$

where the difference is that between the observed and permitted bias and n is the number of specimen pairs minus one.

In the present case

$$t = \frac{(12 - 9.6) \sqrt{9}}{5.10} = \frac{2.4 \sqrt{9}}{5.10} = 1.41.$$

We now look in the t table (Appendix Table 4) under the 10 percent probability level (because the table is two-tailed and we are asking only the one-tailed question Does 12 exceed 9.6?) We find for 9 df the value 1.833, which is greater than the 1.41 we obtained; thus we have not established that 9.6 is smaller than 12 with the requisite confidence. We therefore substitute into the t formula to find the proper value for n, trying out a few values larger than 9. For example, at 15 df the critical t is 1.753. Substituting into the formula,

$$t = \frac{2.4 \sqrt{15}}{5.10} = 1.823.$$

This is larger than 1.753. We therefore need 16 paired analyses to get 15 df, and if the bias and s_d do not change we will have established with 95 percent confidence that 9.6 mg. is an acceptable bias.

In this example we discussed a bias less than that permitted. If the bias were equal to that permitted there would be a 50 percent chance of its being unacceptable, as can be seen from the operating characteristic curves in Figure 21-1; and of course if the bias were greater than that permitted there would be a greater than 50 percent chance of its being unacceptable. Similar deductions could be made regarding the foregoing example on acceptable precision if s equalled or exceeded the s allowed.

Rare Events

One problem which manufacturers generally understand but which certain consumer groups refuse to face is that statistical methods are of little use in predicting rare events. For example, if 1,000 vials of a reagent are tested and meet specifications, is it still possible that the very next vial will be flawed because of some sort of malfunction in the manufacturing process? The answer is obvious; such events do occur, no matter how carefully the process is supervised. Even the best computers are known to make periodic unpredictable errors; this is an unfortunate fact of life. (See Chapter 13.) Fortunately, modern manufacturing processes give rise to very few random accidents; for example, in the CAP Survey Program the millions of vials produced are consistently within the 0.5 percent tolerance specified, although rare accidents do occur.

Current Federal Legislation

The current version of the legislation giving authority to the Food and Drug Administration in the clinical laboratory field is known as the Medical Device Amendments of 1976, Public Law 94-295; this version became law on May 20, 1976. The law has many ramifications, but we will be concerned here with only those facets directly relevant to our statistical discussion.

First, there are labelling requirements which demand provision of specific performance data and other essential information. These data are collected as previously described in Chapter 15. Second, the legislation requires that all devices be classified into one of three categories:

Category I. General controls—require correct labelling.

Category II. Performance standards—must meet certain standards which will ordinarily include accuracy, precision, and freedom from specified interferences. The manufacturer develops data to establish conformance with the standards. If the FDA has reason to doubt this conformance, it may do its own testing using specified techniques. Both of these activities were discussed earlier in this chapter, it being noted that the FDA testing must be much more extensive in many cases to disprove the claims. Many products for common analytes will automatically be considered as "substantially equivalent" to approved products; in that case statistical data may be needed to confirm this equivalency.

Category III. Premarket approval—evidence must be submitted to the FDA and approved by it before the product can be marketed. This requirement will probably not be invoked for many laboratory products, and it has no special statistical connotations.

Information collected and processed as we have described will meet these requirements satisfactorily.

References

1. FDA: GMF: Current good manufacturing practice for medical devices, proposed sections 810.40 (h); 810.60 (C) (2); 810.63; 810.163; 810.169.
2. FDA: GMF: Drugs: Current good manufacturing practice in manufacture, processing, packing or holding: Part 133, Title 121, Code of Federal Regulations, Section 133.11, correction published Federal Register Feb. 4, 1971; 36 FR 2400.

V Statistics in Medical Literature

22 Evaluating Scientific Literature

Scientists keep pace with the rapid advances in their field through reading and attendance at lectures. In both types of educational experience statistics are encountered frequently. For example, the February 9, 1978, issue of the *New England Journal of Medicine* contained a variety of features tabulated in Table 22-1. How does one evaluate the figures that are presented and their meaning?

Almost all the original articles (7 of 8) use some form of statistics, and 5 of the 8 use statistical concepts such as probability or standard deviation.

Assuming that the subject of an article is of sufficient interest to warrant your careful study, you should consider the basic questions discussed below.

Material and Methods

Are material and methods clearly described? The description should include exact references to criteria, to methods used, and to selection of the sample.

Is the sampling appropriate? This refers to proper sample size, completeness, relevance, and random selection.

Was a conscious effort made to avoid sampling bias? The nature of such an effort depends on the type of study. The experimenter should be aware in advance of the potentially destructive consequences if he has foreknowledge of the expected result, whether a chemical value or the response to medication. Somewhere in the article this should be discussed and the precautions described.

Were there outliers, and if so, how were they dealt with?

Results

Are results clearly described and tabulated?
Are results reasonable in light of what is known about the subject?

Statistical Analysis

Is formal statistical analysis necessary or desirable? A cursory glance at the results is often adequate to draw conclusions; statistical analysis is most pertinent when borderline differences are considered, or when the numbers are too large for easy comprehension.

Are the proper formulas used for the type of material presented and the conclusions sought? Common errors are series that are too small; confusion between standard deviation and standard error; and, most annoying, the casual mention of unexplained symbols. For example, "The method is accurate to ± 1 percent" is open to several interpretations—we don't know whether 1 percent includes 1, 2, or 3 coefficients of variation.

Table 22-1
Use of statistics in Feb. 9, 1978 *N. Engl. J. Med.*

Material	Total	Number using statistics	Number using statistical concepts
Major articles	5	4	4
Short articles	3	3	1
Editorials	4	1	0
Case record	1	0	0
Correspondence	31	2	1
	44	10	6

Or "p < .01" is stated without further qualification. The reader knows that the probability has been calculated to be less than .01, but he is not told what events are being compared. For instance, in one study I reviewed, a correct calculation of p less than .0000001 was made. The author properly concluded that the two series being compared were different; he wrongly attributed this to the use of two different test methods, whereas actually it was the patients who were so different.

Are the calculations correct? If the results appear to fit the statistical analysis there is little need to recalculate, but sometimes it is apparent that a mistake must have been made. It is then useful to repeat the calculations.

Conclusions

Are the conclusions applicable to whole populations? One of the commonest mistakes in reasoning is the assumption that a result valid for a sample must therefore apply to larger populations. Even with careful attention to proper random selection and other precautions there may be a hidden difference in groups. This is particularly true for complex organisms such as man, and for small samples.

Are the conclusions justified by the data? All too often careful study of an article leads to the realization that the author jumped "from a preconceived notion to a foregone conclusion," and that the work reported has no bearing on these conclusions. This is particularly true when the field of study involves the interface of science and economics, or science and religion. Although the clinical laboratory is rarely the battleground of religion and science, the conflicts between science and economic gain have become increasingly sharp and this tendency will doubtless intensify.

Examples

We can illustrate some of the problems that arise in the medical use of statistics by reference to current literature:

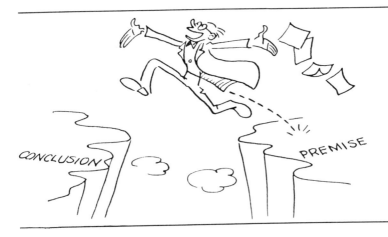

CONCLUSION   PREMISE

Incorrect Calculations: Wrong Formula Employed

The authors [6] treated 10 patients suffering from benign prostatic hypertrophy with a drug, and 6 were improved, by their criteria; of 10 controls equally afflicted but not receiving the drug, only 2 improved. The authors write, "A chi-square test was highly significant (p < .005)." Offhand this seems unlikely, so we recalculate using the formula in Chapter 4. Our chi-square result is 1.87, which is not significant at even p = .10 for 1 df. The calculations in the article were therefore wrong. Additionally, we know that for small series a 2 × 2 contingency table for unequal samples (Appendix Table 5) is the proper tool. In such a table we look under $A = 10$, $B = 10$, $a = 6$, and we find that the significant level of b at 0.05 is 1; 2 is therefore not significant. This confirms our suspicion of incorrect calculation.

Failure to Perform Statistical Test

The author [9] quotes his control series of 2,335 patients who had been operated on, and of whom 28 died of perioperative cardiopulmonary arrest. Of these 25 were autopsied, and of these 17 had necropsy-confirmed evidence of death due to thromboembolism. His new series, treated with preoperative heparin, consisted of 565 patients; 2 died of cardiopulmonary arrest, neither of thromboembolism. He concludes that his treatment prevents thromboembolism, but he does not calculate the statistical verification of this.

This is a standard chi-square problem, but we are at a loss to know how to substitute in the formula

$$\chi^2 = \frac{n\left(\left|ad - bc\right| - \frac{n}{2}\right)^2}{(a + b)(c + d)(a + c)(b + d)}$$

If we compare death rate only, our table is $a = 28$, $b = 2$, $c = 2{,}307$, $d = 563$, and χ^2 is 2.40, which is not significant. If we compare death rate due to proven thromboembolic disease our table is $a = 17, b = 0, c = 2,318, d = 565$, and χ^2 becomes 3.08, which is also not significant at p = .05. Finally, if we compare all 28 deaths in the first series with 0 in the experimental series our table is $a = 28$, $b = 0, c = 2,307$, and $d = 565$.

The χ^2 value is now 5.65, which is significant at the 0.975 probability level. This is statistically significant but the reasoning is incorrect. This example points out the potential value of statistical thinking in making the problem itself clear.

Effective and Sophisticated Use of Statistics

The investigators [2] performed an evaluation of a large automated device used for hematology testing. Reproducibility of individual values is reported as standard deviation and coefficient of variation and is carried out on large numbers of samples. Patient comparisons are performed on a large series using specified and reliable conventional methods. The number of tests performed by each method, the details of each method, and the experimental design are clearly defined. Reliance on properly paired results creates meaningful statistics.

In comparing performance the authors use the formula

$$CV = \frac{\sigma}{\bar{x}} = \frac{\sqrt{\frac{\Sigma d^2}{2n}}}{\bar{x}}$$

to calculate the coefficient of variation of the difference between methods. This differs from the formulas we recommend for s which are

$$s = \sqrt{\frac{\Sigma d^2}{n - 1}}$$

and

$$CV = \frac{100\ s}{\bar{x}}$$

The use of σ rather than s is not correct because σ refers to true population standard deviation, which is not known, whereas s is the standard deviation found by experiment. Use of $2n$ rather than $n - 1$ in the denominator is valid because the authors have not subtracted the bias, which we did; therefore the difference between two determinations, each with its own imprecision, is greater than that between single values and the mean difference and requires a larger divisor. Omission of the 100 multiplier in the formula was inadvertent, and the calculations were actually performed correctly.

Table 22-2
Effect of Chocolate on Acne: 65 Patients*

Condition	Control Bar	Chocolate Bar
Worse	7	9
Same	53	46
Improved	5	10

*Data from Fulton, Plewig, and Kligman [5].

Simple Data, Clear Presentation: Statistical Analysis Not Needed

The physicians [5] were interested in the effect of eating chocolate on the lesions of acne vulgaris. They performed a single blind crossover experiment. Bars were prepared which were either chocolate or a substitute that allegedly tasted exactly the same. The subjects ate one type of bar for four weeks, ate neither type for three weeks, and then ate the other type for four weeks. Choice of which bar was consumed first was presumably randomized. Lesions were counted; therefore findings of the examiner were objective and a double-blind format was unnecessary. The results are put in a neat bar graph; for our purposes they may be tabulated for the 65 patients who participated, as shown in Table 22-2. A quick glance indicates that these results are essentially the same, and no statistical analysis is needed.

Controversy About Basic Data

The investigators [11] commented on an earlier paper purporting to show that a certain drug was associated with an increased incidence of gastrointestinal bleeding in 32 patients. They claimed to have reviewed the original patient records and to have discovered the following:

1. 4 charts could not be found.
2. 12 patients had gastrointestinal bleeding before the drug was given.
3. 14 patients bled after the drug was given; but other diseases and treatments, all noted in the records, could well have caused the bleeding.

The authors conclude that no association of the drug and the bleeding was established.

The authors of the original article provide their rebuttal. They point out:

1. They found the missing charts easily.
2. Their data were based on a drug surveillance system not recorded in patients' routine charts and claimed to be much more accurate than these charts.
3. There was often doubt as to the time sequences of drug administration and bleeding episodes.

This sort of controversy is very useful because it is in the original data that most trouble arises. Recourse to original data is often difficult and time-consuming, but if the problem is critical there may be no alternative way to check the results.

Correct Use of Chi-square: Failure to Subject Appropriate
Data to Statistical Analysis

The medical attendants [10] observe that hypothermia is common in hypo-glycemic states but rare in other conditions which produce similar clinical manifestations. They find 8 of 15 hypoglycemic patients, and 1 of 20 clinically similar patients with normal or elevated blood glucose, to have subnormal temperatures.

They claim a highly significant difference between the two groups, χ^2 = 8.105, $p < 0.01$. We recalculate and find this is correct. They then mention that all 5 subjects first seen between 5 A.M. and noon were hypothermic, but only 3 of 10 seen at other hours were hypothermic; they do not attempt statistical analysis. Because there are too few cases for chi-square study we go to Appendix Table 5. A must exceed B, so we reverse the question to read as follows: What are the chances that 7 of 10 negatives are from the same population as 0 of 5? In our table, then, $A = 10$, $a = 7$, $B = 5$. The b value is listed as 0.019; i.e., significant at .05 level two-tailed.

The authors could thereby have claimed statistical significance for the observation that morning hypothermia is more reliable than afternoon hypothermia in diagnosing hypoglycemia.

Hazards of Comparing Incidence of Disease in Different Series

The investigators [8] were interested in a prior observation that there was an association between salivary gland cancer and breast cancer. In their own material, comprising twice as many cases as the first series, they found no such association. The importance of this study lies in the authors' comments, one of which we quote: "A very cogent and apropos appraisal of such methods was presented by Epstein, who showed that by comparing his figures to the data of different registries he could prove that the incidence of second primary cancers was greater than, less than, or the same as the incidence expected by chance alone."*

Again we face the sampling problem: Do the samples really represent the same population?

---

*This is a good place to comment briefly on appraising an article by looking at its source. This particular item is from the Mayo Clinic, which has had a strong medical statistics department for many years. Elvebach is a sound and experienced member of this department, so the views expressed should be taken very seriously. If authors are unknown or known to be unsophisticated in the field their opinions should be viewed more cautiously.

Conclusions Unsupported by the Data

Amador and Hsi [1] in an interesting and comprehensive analysis compare normal ranges derived from healthy persons with normal ranges derived from patient studies by six indirect methods. They found that for the six tests studied there was poor correspondence between ranges obtained from normal persons (35 to 110 subjects) and the ranges calculated by indirect methods. For most tests the means were appreciably higher by the indirect techniques. They conclude, "The indirect estimates based on test results from adult hospital patients were quite inaccurate because the estimated means were shifted significantly toward pathologic values and the estimated standard deviations were unacceptably wide." They also state, "For an indirect method to be acceptable, however, it must yield the same range as that obtained by the same assay method in the same laboratory on healthy subjects for all common laboratory tests."

There is no problem in accepting the fact that the methods based on patient values are different from those based on healthy, normal persons. The data presented are straightforward, the statistics are valid, and the observations are in accord with common experience. The real problem lies in the second sentence quoted above. If this definition of *acceptable* is correct, then indeed the indirect methods are inaccurate. If, however, we admit that hospital patients are inevitably a different population than are healthy persons, that being sick in a hospital automatically changes certain chemical blood values, and that we wish to compare individual patients with their own peer group, i.e., other hospital patients, we could equally well have concluded from the facts presented that the direct estimations of normal values were inaccurate because they differed from those of hospital patients!

Certainly we cannot solve this problem, which is philosophic rather than statistical; we merely point out that statistics cannot answer the question of Which is the correct range for our patient? The conclusions drawn are foregone and not warranted by the data.

Presentation of Selected Data: Inadequate Statistical Analysis

The authors [12] present their experience with a novel device for separating plasma without centrifugation. The only data presented are for six paired samples "in the largest single comparative experiment"; values are presented for blood samples from which plasma was separated by conventional means and by the new method. From the data, without statistics of any kind, they conclude that for many components the results are "essentially equivalent" but for others there was a significant difference.

The criticisms of this work are obvious. A single experiment with six paired samples is insufficient to support the thesis that results are essentially equivalent; particularly it fails to consider the possibility that certain plasmas may give very different results by the two techniques. If further studies were done, which seems likely from the discussion, why aren't they tabulated or summarized? This article then falls far short of presenting in proper form the comparative data recommended in Chapter 15, Choice of Methods, and is inadequate to establish its thesis.

Additionally, use of so-called typical, representative, or selected data must always be suspect. It may very likely have been chosen because it is typical of what the authors would like to demonstrate, rather than typical of what actually occurred.

Confusing Use of SE Instead of SD

In recommending the use of the ratio of amylase clearance to creatinine clearance for differential diagnosis, the authors [7] publish a table of the ratios in normal controls, hospitalized patients, persons with pancreatitis of various durations, and several other groups. The means of each series with the SE is given; for example, hospital controls are 3.1 ± 0.3, and pancreatitis (0–4 days) patients are 6.6 ± 0.3. Many readers, interested in diagnosis, would conclude that this test provides quite an infallible separation of the two groups. However, in a subsequent bar graph one can observe overlap in the two groups. Because clinicians use tests to diagnose individual patients rather than groups, the relevant figure diagnostically is the SD. Recalculated as SD, by multiplying the SE by the square root of n for each series, the comparison of 3.1 ± 1.27 with 6.6 ± 1.70 would have given a truer picture and would have predicted the overlap found. Feinstein has recently condemned the practice of using SE inappropriately in an extensive polemic [4].

Most articles using statistics pose problems similar to those presented in the examples given, so there is no reason to give further instances. I am confident that every reader will find other examples with no difficulty!

References

1. Amador, E., and Hsi, B. P. Indirect methods for estimating the normal range. *Am. J. Clin. Pathol.* 52:538–546, 1969.
2. Brittin, G. M., Brecher, G., and Johnson, C. A. Evaluation of the Coulter Counter Model S. *Am. J. Clin. Pathol.* 52:679–689, 1969.
3. Brittin, G. M., Brecher, G., Johnson, C. A., and Elashoff, R. M. Stability of blood in commonly used anticoagulants: Use of refrigerated blood for quality control of the Coulter Counter Model S. *Am. J. Clin. Pathol.* 52:690–694, 1969.
4. Feinstein, A. R. Clinical biostatistics XXXVII. *Clin. Pharmacol. Ther.* 20:617–631, 1976.
5. Fulton, J. E., Jr., Plewig, G., and Kligman, A. M. Effect of chocolate on acne vulgaris. *J.A.M.A.* 210:2071–2074, 1969.
6. Geller, J., Angrist, A., Nakao, K., and Newman, H. Therapy with progestational agents in advanced benign prostatic hypertrophy. *J.A.M.A.* 210:1421–1427, 1969.
7. Levitt, M. D., Rapoport, M., and Cooperband, S. R. The renal clearance of amylase in renal insufficiency, acute pancreatitis and macroamylasemia. *Ann. Intern. Med.* 71:919–925, 1969.

8. Moertel, C. G., and Elvebach, L. R. The association between salivary gland cancer and breast cancer. *J.A.M.A.* 210:306–308, 1969.
9. Sharnoff, J. G. Prevention of sudden cardiopulmonary arrest in the perioperative period with prophylactic heparin. *Lancet* 2:292–293, 1969.
10. Strauch, B. S., Felig, P., Baxter, J. D., and Schimpf, S. C. Hypothermia in hypoglycemia. *J.A.M.A.* 210:345–346, 1969.
11. Wilkinson, W. H., Ciminera, J. L., and Simpkins, G. T. Intravenously given ethacrynic acid and gastrointestinal bleeding: Letter to editor. *J.A.M.A.* 210:34, 1969. Reply by D. Slone, H. Jick, G. P. Lewis, S. Shapiro, and O. S. Miettinen, ibid.
12. Winkelman, J., and Pileggi, V. J. Clinical chemistry testing on plasma obtained without centrifugation. *Am. J. Clin. Pathol.* 52:623–626, 1969.

23 Presenting Statistical Data

In the last chapter we discussed scientific presentations from the point of view of the consumer. Because most laboratory specialists at some time become authors or lecturers, this chapter is devoted to the problems of the producer.

When statistical data are used in scientific presentations, much of the impact of the data is often lost because the writer or lecturer is so concerned with his own problems that he neglects the audience. The following are a few guidelines which, although self-evident, are commonly ignored.

General Principles

The nature of the raw material should be clearly explained. Too often the author assumes that his intimate knowledge of the original data is shared by everyone. A clear definition of the population and how the sample was chosen should appear early in any presentation.

Precautions taken to avoid sampling error should be discussed. Good, statistically oriented thinking requires constant attention to proper sampling. The nature of the precautions used is of great interest to anyone analyzing the data.

Statistical terms should be defined. The author cannot assume that statistical terms and usage are so familiar that no explanation is necessary. Furthermore, there are different ways of presenting the data, all acceptable, but each requiring interpretation. If there are alternative methods of calculation the pertinent formula should be displayed. If a complicated or unfamiliar mathematical manipulation is involved a sample calculation is imperative.

Consistency of usage is desirable. All the figures in each table should be carried out to the same number of significant places and should be expressed in the same units.

Graphs are extremely valuable if they are properly planned. Both line and bar graphs provide excellent visual impact. Unfortunately this may be blunted by one of the common flaws listed here. Almost all these errors arise from an attempt to put too much data on a single graph. The proper goal is "instant comprehension," and several small, clear graphs, each making a single point, are much superior to a single large, confusing graph. Avoid these errors:

1. *Intersecting lines.* A series of wandering "squiggles" which cannot be separated quickly by the eye are commonly presented; they are useless.
2. *Subdivided bars.* In bar graphs the eye is caught by the relative height of the bars. If each is further subdivided by color or cross-hatching, and if there are numerous bars, the observer loses his way quickly.
3. *Figures too small.* When an effort is made to provide excessive data the labels and figures are often too small to be legible.

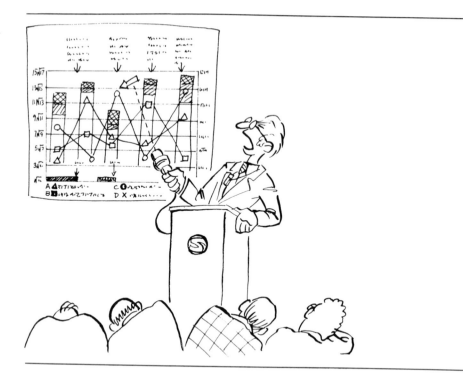

4. *Confusing symbols*. Sometimes a graph is filled with open circles, closed circles, triangles, stars, and so on. Unless they are large enough to be readily recognized, and unless they form clear-cut patterns, they are confusing.

Written Publications

Raw data should be as complete as possible. This often involves a compromise between the desire of the author to give all the figures and the ability of the journal to publish masses of material. Frequently the raw data can be manipulated in different ways to unearth hidden meanings; if only a summary is presented, the reader is unable to try these diverse approaches.

Good summary tables are essential. These tables should be self-explanatory and should bear a clear and complete caption. A complex table annotated "Refer to the text for explanation" will rarely be studied. The number of categories should be small enough so that each entry is clearly legible.

Oral Presentations

Oral presentations require that the statistical information be displayed either by slides or on a blackboard. Although the manner of the physical presentation may seem a minor point unworthy of the scholarly nature of this book, so many excellent talks are ruined by small disasters that I feel no compunction about discussing these problems.

The figures must be legible. This means that tables should be limited to the minimum number of entries. Radiomats, which provide about 13 lines of type, each about 33 spaces across, are cheap and useful; slides with more entries than this cannot be read easily in the average auditorium. 3¼ × 4 slides are a nuisance to transport but are usually projected better than are the more common 35 mm. transparencies.

Graphs should be simple and clear. This is as important as with published graphs because they must be displayed quickly and are not available for prolonged study.

The amount of data must be limited. Unless the presentation is a long one there is no time for illustrating masses of raw data. Effective summaries are much better.

Leave the slides on long enough so that they can be read and comprehended. This requires that the lecturer realistically limit the material he wishes to present. Each slide should be explained clearly while it is on display to provide a simultaneous visual and auditory exposition.

If possible, the auditorium should be partly lighted. This permits interested listeners to make notes about the data. Slides illustrating tables or graphs can usually be read adequately without total darkness.

If these relatively simple hints are followed the level of scientific data presentation will be substantially improved.

Appendix Tables

Appendix Table 1
Random Number Table

49	54	43	54	82		17	37	93	23	78		87	35	20	96	43		84	26	34	91	64
57	24	55	06	88		77	04	74	47	67		21	76	33	50	25		83	92	12	06	76
16	95	55	67	19		98	10	50	71	75		12	86	73	58	07		44	39	52	38	79
78	64	56	07	82		52	42	07	44	38		15	51	00	13	42		99	66	02	79	54
09	47	27	96	54		49	17	46	09	62		90	52	84	77	27		08	02	73	43	28
44	17	16	58	09		79	83	86	19	62		06	76	50	03	10		55	23	64	05	05
84	16	07	44	99		83	11	46	32	24		20	14	85	88	45		10	93	72	88	71
82	97	77	77	81		07	45	32	14	08		32	98	94	07	72		93	85	79	10	75
50	92	26	11	97		00	56	76	31	38		80	22	02	53	53		86	60	42	04	53
83	39	50	08	30		42	34	07	96	88		54	42	06	87	98		35	85	29	48	39
40	33	20	38	26		13	89	51	03	74		17	76	37	13	04		07	74	21	19	30
96	83	50	87	75		97	12	25	93	47		70	33	24	03	54		97	77	46	44	80
88	42	95	45	72		16	64	36	16	00		04	43	18	66	79		94	77	24	21	90
33	27	14	34	09		45	59	34	68	49		12	72	07	34	45		99	27	72	95	14
50	27	89	87	19		20	15	37	00	49		52	85	66	60	44		38	68	88	11	80
55	74	30	77	40		44	22	78	84	26		04	33	46	09	52		68	07	97	06	57
59	29	97	68	60		71	91	38	67	54		13	58	18	24	76		15	54	55	95	52
48	55	90	65	72		96	57	69	36	10		96	46	92	42	45		97	60	49	04	91
66	37	32	20	30		77	84	57	03	29		10	45	65	04	26		11	04	96	67	24
68	49	69	10	82		53	75	91	93	30		34	25	20	57	27		40	48	73	51	92
83	62	64	11	12		67	19	00	71	74		60	47	21	29	68		02	02	37	03	31
06	09	19	74	66		02	94	37	34	02		76	70	90	30	86		38	45	94	30	38
33	32	51	26	38		79	78	45	04	91		16	92	53	56	16		02	75	50	95	98
42	38	97	01	50		87	75	66	81	41		40	01	74	91	62		48	51	84	08	32
96	44	33	49	13		34	86	82	53	91		00	52	43	48	85		27	55	26	89	62
64	05	71	95	86		11	05	65	09	68		76	83	20	37	90		57	16	00	11	66
75	73	88	05	90		52	27	41	14	86		22	98	12	22	08		07	52	74	95	80
33	96	02	75	19		07	60	62	93	55		59	33	82	43	90		49	37	38	44	59
97	51	40	14	02		04	02	33	31	08		39	54	16	49	36		47	95	93	13	30
15	06	15	93	20		01	90	10	75	06		40	78	78	89	62		02	67	74	17	33
22	35	85	15	13		92	03	51	59	77		59	56	78	06	83		52	91	05	70	74
09	98	42	99	64		61	71	62	99	15		06	51	29	16	93		58	05	77	09	51
54	87	66	47	54		73	32	08	11	12		44	95	92	63	16		29	56	24	29	48
58	37	78	80	70		42	10	50	67	42		32	17	55	85	74		94	44	67	16	94
87	59	36	22	41		26	78	63	06	55		13	08	27	01	50		15	29	39	39	43
71	41	61	50	72		12	41	94	96	26		44	95	27	36	99		02	96	74	30	83
23	52	23	33	12		96	93	02	18	39		07	02	18	36	07		25	99	32	70	23
31	04	49	69	96		10	47	48	45	88		13	41	43	89	20		97	17	14	49	17
31	99	73	68	68		35	81	33	03	76		24	30	12	48	60		18	99	10	72	34
94	58	28	41	36		45	37	59	03	09		90	35	57	29	12		82	62	54	65	60
98	80	33	00	91		09	77	93	19	82		74	94	80	04	04		45	07	31	66	49
73	81	53	94	79		33	62	46	86	28		08	31	54	46	31		53	94	13	38	47
73	82	97	22	21		05	03	27	24	83		72	89	44	05	60		35	80	39	94	88
22	95	75	42	49		39	32	82	22	49		02	48	07	70	37		16	04	61	67	87
39	00	03	06	90		55	85	78	38	36		94	37	30	69	32		90	89	00	76	33

Source: W. J. Youden, *Statistical Techniques for Collaborative Tests* (Washington, D.C.: Association of Official Analytical Chemists, 1967).
Text Explanation: pages 8, 63, 64.

Appendix Table 2
F Distribution, Upper 5 Percent Points (F .95)

Degrees of Freedom for Numerator

v_2 \ v_1	1	2	3	4	5	6	7	8	9	10	12	15	20	24	30	40	60	120	∞
1	161.4	199.5	215.7	224.6	230.2	234.0	236.8	238.9	240.5	241.9	243.9	245.9	248.0	249.1	250.1	251.1	252.2	253.3	254.3
2	18.51	19.00	19.16	19.25	19.30	19.33	19.35	19.37	19.38	19.40	19.41	19.43	19.45	19.45	19.46	19.47	19.48	19.49	19.50
3	10.13	9.55	9.28	9.12	9.01	8.94	8.89	8.85	8.81	8.79	8.74	8.70	8.66	8.64	8.62	8.59	8.57	8.55	8.53
4	7.71	6.94	6.59	6.39	6.26	6.16	6.09	6.04	6.00	5.96	5.91	5.86	5.80	5.77	5.75	5.72	5.69	5.66	5.63
5	6.61	5.79	5.41	5.19	5.05	4.95	4.88	4.82	4.77	4.74	4.68	4.62	4.56	4.53	4.50	4.46	4.43	4.40	4.36
6	5.99	5.14	4.76	4.53	4.39	4.28	4.21	4.15	4.10	4.06	4.00	3.94	3.87	3.84	3.81	3.77	3.74	3.70	3.67
7	5.59	4.74	4.35	4.12	3.97	3.87	3.79	3.73	3.68	3.64	3.57	3.51	3.44	3.41	3.38	3.34	3.30	3.27	3.23
8	5.32	4.46	4.07	3.84	3.69	3.58	3.50	3.44	3.39	3.35	3.28	3.22	3.15	3.12	3.08	3.04	3.01	2.97	2.93
9	5.12	4.26	3.86	3.63	3.48	3.37	3.29	3.23	3.18	3.14	3.07	3.01	2.94	2.90	2.86	2.83	2.79	2.75	2.71
10	4.96	4.10	3.71	3.48	3.33	3.22	3.14	3.07	3.02	2.98	2.91	2.85	2.77	2.74	2.70	2.66	2.62	2.58	2.54
11	4.84	3.98	3.59	3.36	3.20	3.09	3.01	2.95	2.90	2.85	2.79	2.72	2.65	2.61	2.57	2.53	2.49	2.45	2.40
12	4.75	3.89	3.49	3.26	3.11	3.00	2.91	2.85	2.80	2.75	2.69	2.62	2.54	2.51	2.47	2.43	2.38	2.34	2.30
13	4.67	3.81	3.41	3.18	3.03	2.92	2.83	2.77	2.71	2.67	2.60	2.53	2.46	2.42	2.38	2.34	2.30	2.25	2.21
14	4.60	3.74	3.34	3.11	2.96	2.85	2.76	2.70	2.65	2.60	2.53	2.46	2.39	2.35	2.31	2.27	2.22	2.18	2.13
15	4.54	3.68	3.29	3.06	2.90	2.79	2.71	2.64	2.59	2.54	2.48	2.40	2.33	2.29	2.25	2.20	2.16	2.11	2.07
16	4.49	3.63	3.24	3.01	2.85	2.74	2.66	2.59	2.54	2.49	2.42	2.35	2.28	2.24	2.19	2.15	2.11	2.06	2.01
17	4.45	3.59	3.20	2.96	2.81	2.70	2.61	2.55	2.49	2.45	2.38	2.31	2.23	2.19	2.15	2.10	2.06	2.01	1.96
18	4.41	3.55	3.16	2.93	2.77	2.66	2.58	2.51	2.46	2.41	2.34	2.27	2.19	2.15	2.11	2.06	2.02	1.97	1.92
19	4.38	3.52	3.13	2.90	2.74	2.63	2.54	2.48	2.42	2.38	2.31	2.23	2.16	2.11	2.07	2.03	1.98	1.93	1.88
20	4.35	3.49	3.10	2.87	2.71	2.60	2.51	2.45	2.39	2.35	2.28	2.20	2.12	2.08	2.04	1.99	1.95	1.90	1.84
21	4.32	3.47	3.07	2.84	2.68	2.57	2.49	2.42	2.37	2.32	2.25	2.18	2.10	2.05	2.01	1.96	1.92	1.87	1.81
22	4.30	3.44	3.05	2.82	2.66	2.55	2.46	2.40	2.34	2.30	2.23	2.15	2.07	2.03	1.98	1.94	1.89	1.84	1.78
23	4.28	3.42	3.03	2.80	2.64	2.53	2.44	2.37	2.32	2.27	2.20	2.13	2.05	2.01	1.96	1.91	1.86	1.81	1.76
24	4.26	3.40	3.01	2.78	2.62	2.51	2.42	2.36	2.30	2.25	2.18	2.11	2.03	1.98	1.94	1.89	1.84	1.79	1.73
25	4.24	3.39	2.99	2.76	2.60	2.49	2.40	2.34	2.28	2.24	2.16	2.09	2.01	1.96	1.92	1.87	1.82	1.77	1.71
26	4.23	3.37	2.98	2.74	2.59	2.47	2.39	2.32	2.27	2.22	2.15	2.07	1.99	1.95	1.90	1.85	1.80	1.75	1.69
27	4.21	3.35	2.96	2.73	2.57	2.46	2.37	2.31	2.25	2.20	2.13	2.06	1.97	1.93	1.88	1.84	1.79	1.73	1.67
28	4.20	3.34	2.95	2.71	2.56	2.45	2.36	2.29	2.24	2.19	2.12	2.04	1.96	1.91	1.87	1.82	1.77	1.71	1.65
29	4.18	3.33	2.93	2.70	2.55	2.43	2.35	2.28	2.22	2.18	2.10	2.03	1.94	1.90	1.85	1.81	1.75	1.70	1.64
30	4.17	3.32	2.92	2.69	2.53	2.42	2.33	2.27	2.21	2.16	2.09	2.01	1.93	1.89	1.84	1.79	1.74	1.68	1.62
40	4.08	3.23	2.84	2.61	2.45	2.34	2.25	2.18	2.12	2.08	2.00	1.92	1.84	1.79	1.74	1.69	1.64	1.58	1.51
60	4.00	3.15	2.76	2.53	2.37	2.25	2.17	2.10	2.04	1.99	1.92	1.84	1.75	1.70	1.65	1.59	1.53	1.47	1.39
120	3.92	3.07	2.68	2.45	2.29	2.17	2.09	2.02	1.96	1.91	1.83	1.75	1.66	1.61	1.55	1.50	1.43	1.35	1.25
∞	3.84	3.00	2.60	2.37	2.21	2.10	2.01	1.94	1.88	1.83	1.75	1.67	1.57	1.52	1.46	1.39	1.32	1.22	1.00

Degrees of Freedom for Denominator

$F = \dfrac{s_1^2}{s_2^2} = \dfrac{S_1/v_1}{S_2/v_2}$, where $s_1^2 = S_1/v_1$ and $s_2^2 = S_2/v_2$ are independent mean squares estimating a common variance σ^2 and based on v_1 and v_2 degrees of freedom, respectively.

Note: Interpolation should be performed using reciprocals of the degrees of freedom.

Source: E. S. Pearson and H. O. Hartley (Eds.), *Biometrika Tables for Statisticians* (3rd ed.) (Cambridge, England: Cambridge University Press, 1966), Table 18.

Text Explanation: pages 8, 17, 25, 26.

Appendix Table 5
F Distribution, Upper 1 Percent Points (F .99)

Degrees of Freedom for Numerator

$\nu_2 \backslash \nu_1$	1	2	3	4	5	6	7	8	9	10	12	15	20	24	30	40	60	120	∞
1	4052	4999.5	5403	5625	5764	5859	5928	5981	6022	6056	6106	6157	6209	6235	6261	6287	6313	6339	6366
2	98.50	99.00	99.17	99.25	99.30	99.33	99.36	99.37	99.39	99.40	99.42	99.43	99.45	99.46	99.47	99.47	99.48	99.49	99.50
3	34.12	30.82	29.46	28.71	28.24	27.91	27.67	27.49	27.35	27.23	27.05	26.87	26.69	26.60	26.50	26.41	26.32	26.22	26.13
4	21.20	18.00	16.69	15.98	15.52	15.21	14.98	14.80	14.66	14.55	14.37	14.20	14.02	13.93	13.84	13.75	13.65	13.56	13.46
5	16.26	13.27	12.06	11.39	10.97	10.67	10.46	10.29	10.16	10.05	9.89	9.72	9.55	9.47	9.38	9.29	9.20	9.11	9.02
6	13.75	10.92	9.78	9.15	8.75	8.47	8.26	8.10	7.98	7.87	7.72	7.56	7.40	7.31	7.23	7.14	7.06	6.97	6.88
7	12.25	9.55	8.45	7.85	7.46	7.19	6.99	6.84	6.72	6.62	6.47	6.31	6.16	6.07	5.99	5.91	5.82	5.74	5.65
8	11.26	8.65	7.59	7.01	6.63	6.37	6.18	6.03	5.91	5.81	5.67	5.52	5.36	5.28	5.20	5.12	5.03	4.95	4.86
9	10.56	8.02	6.99	6.42	6.06	5.80	5.61	5.47	5.35	5.26	5.11	4.96	4.81	4.73	4.65	4.57	4.48	4.40	4.31
10	10.04	7.56	6.55	5.99	5.64	5.39	5.20	5.06	4.94	4.85	4.71	4.56	4.41	4.33	4.25	4.17	4.08	4.00	3.91
11	9.65	7.21	6.22	5.67	5.32	5.07	4.89	4.74	4.63	4.54	4.40	4.25	4.10	4.02	3.94	3.86	3.78	3.69	3.60
12	9.33	6.93	5.95	5.41	5.06	4.82	4.64	4.50	4.39	4.30	4.16	4.01	3.86	3.78	3.70	3.62	3.54	3.45	3.36
13	9.07	6.70	5.74	5.21	4.86	4.62	4.44	4.30	4.19	4.10	3.96	3.82	3.66	3.59	3.51	3.43	3.34	3.25	3.17
14	8.86	6.51	5.56	5.04	4.69	4.46	4.28	4.14	4.03	3.94	3.80	3.66	3.51	3.43	3.35	3.27	3.18	3.09	3.00
15	8.68	6.36	5.42	4.89	4.56	4.32	4.14	4.00	3.89	3.80	3.67	3.52	3.37	3.29	3.21	3.13	3.05	2.96	2.87
16	8.53	6.23	5.29	4.77	4.44	4.20	4.03	3.89	3.78	3.69	3.55	3.41	3.26	3.18	3.10	3.02	2.93	2.84	2.75
17	8.40	6.11	5.18	4.67	4.34	4.10	3.93	3.79	3.68	3.59	3.46	3.31	3.16	3.08	3.00	2.92	2.83	2.75	2.65
18	8.29	6.01	5.09	4.58	4.25	4.01	3.84	3.71	3.60	3.51	3.37	3.23	3.08	3.00	2.92	2.84	2.75	2.66	2.57
19	8.18	5.93	5.01	4.50	4.17	3.94	3.77	3.63	3.52	3.43	3.30	3.15	3.00	2.92	2.84	2.76	2.67	2.58	2.49
20	8.10	5.85	4.94	4.43	4.10	3.87	3.70	3.56	3.46	3.37	3.23	3.09	2.94	2.86	2.78	2.69	2.61	2.52	2.42
21	8.02	5.78	4.87	4.37	4.04	3.81	3.64	3.51	3.40	3.31	3.17	3.03	2.88	2.80	2.72	2.64	2.55	2.46	2.36
22	7.95	5.72	4.82	4.31	3.99	3.76	3.59	3.45	3.35	3.26	3.12	2.98	2.83	2.75	2.67	2.58	2.50	2.40	2.31
23	7.88	5.66	4.76	4.26	3.94	3.71	3.54	3.41	3.30	3.21	3.07	2.93	2.78	2.70	2.62	2.54	2.45	2.35	2.26
24	7.82	5.61	4.72	4.22	3.90	3.67	3.50	3.36	3.26	3.17	3.03	2.89	2.74	2.66	2.58	2.49	2.40	2.31	2.21
25	7.77	5.57	4.68	4.18	3.85	3.63	3.46	3.32	3.22	3.13	2.99	2.85	2.70	2.62	2.54	2.45	2.36	2.27	2.17
26	7.72	5.53	4.64	4.14	3.82	3.59	3.42	3.29	3.18	3.09	2.96	2.81	2.66	2.58	2.50	2.42	2.33	2.23	2.13
27	7.68	5.49	4.60	4.11	3.78	3.56	3.39	3.26	3.15	3.06	2.93	2.78	2.63	2.55	2.47	2.38	2.29	2.20	2.10
28	7.64	5.45	4.57	4.07	3.75	3.53	3.36	3.23	3.12	3.03	2.90	2.75	2.60	2.52	2.44	2.35	2.26	2.17	2.06
29	7.60	5.42	4.54	4.04	3.73	3.50	3.33	3.20	3.09	3.00	2.87	2.73	2.57	2.49	2.41	2.33	2.23	2.14	2.03
30	7.56	5.39	4.51	4.02	3.70	3.47	3.30	3.17	3.07	2.98	2.84	2.70	2.55	2.47	2.39	2.30	2.21	2.11	2.01
40	7.31	5.18	4.31	3.83	3.51	3.29	3.12	2.99	2.89	2.80	2.66	2.52	2.37	2.29	2.20	2.11	2.02	1.92	1.80
60	7.08	4.98	4.13	3.65	3.34	3.12	2.95	2.82	2.72	2.63	2.50	2.35	2.20	2.12	2.03	1.94	1.84	1.73	1.60
120	6.85	4.79	3.95	3.48	3.17	2.96	2.79	2.66	2.56	2.47	2.34	2.19	2.03	1.95	1.86	1.76	1.66	1.53	1.38
∞	6.63	4.61	3.78	3.32	3.02	2.80	2.64	2.51	2.41	2.32	2.18	2.04	1.88	1.79	1.70	1.59	1.47	1.32	1.00

Degrees of Freedom for Denominator

$r = \dfrac{s_1^2}{s_2^2} = \dfrac{S_1/\nu_1}{S_2/\nu_2}$, where $s_1^2 = S_1/\nu_1$ and $s_2^2 = S_2/\nu_2$ are independent mean squares estimating a common variance σ^2 and based on ν_1 and ν_2 degrees of freedom, respectively.

Note: Interpolation should be performed using reciprocals of the degrees of freedom.
Source: E. S. Pearson and H. O. Hartley (Eds.), *Biometrika Tables for Statisticians* (3d ed.) (Cambridge, England: Cambridge University Press, 1966). Table 18.
Text Explanation: pages 8, 17, 25, 26.

Appendix Table 4
Critical Values of *t*

df	\multicolumn{7}{c}{Percent Probability Level}						
	50	40	30	20	10	5	1
1	1.000	1.376	1.963	3.078	6.314	12.706	63.657
2	.816	1.061	1.386	1.886	2.920	4.303	9.925
3	.765	.978	1.250	1.638	2.353	3.182	5.841
4	.741	.941	1.190	1.533	2.132	2.776	4.604
5	.727	.920	1.156	1.476	2.015	2.571	4.032
6	.718	.906	1.134	1.440	1.943	2.447	3.707
7	.711	.896	1.119	1.415	1.895	2.365	3.499
8	.706	.889	1.108	1.397	1.860	2.306	3.355
9	.703	.883	1.100	1.383	1.833	2.262	3.250
10	.700	.879	1.093	1.372	1.812	2.228	3.169
11	.697	.876	1.088	1.363	1.796	2.201	3.106
12	.695	.873	1.083	1.356	1.782	2.179	3.055
13	.694	.870	1.079	1.350	1.771	2.160	3.012
14	.692	.868	1.076	1.345	1.761	2.145	2.977
15	.691	.866	1.074	1.341	1.753	2.131	2.947
16	.690	.865	1.071	1.337	1.746	2.120	2.921
17	.689	.863	1.069	1.333	1.740	2.110	2.898
18	.688	.862	1.067	1.330	1.734	2.101	2.878
19	.688	.861	1.066	1.328	1.729	2.093	2.861
20	.687	.860	1.064	1.325	1.725	2.086	2.845
21	.686	.859	1.063	1.323	1.721	2.080	2.831
22	.686	.858	1.061	1.321	1.717	2.074	2.819
23	.685	.858	1.060	1.319	1.714	2.069	2.807
24	.685	.857	1.059	1.318	1.711	2.064	2.797
25	.684	.856	1.058	1.316	1.708	2.060	2.787
26	.684	.856	1.058	1.315	1.706	2.056	2.779
27	.684	.855	1.057	1.314	1.703	2.052	2.771
28	.683	.855	1.056	1.313	1.701	2.048	2.763
29	.683	.854	1.055	1.311	1.699	2.045	2.756
30	.683	.854	1.055	1.310	1.697	2.042	2.750
40	.681	.851	1.050	1.303	1.684	2.021	2.704
50	.680	.849	1.048	1.299	1.676	2.008	2.678
60	.679	.848	1.046	1.296	1.671	2.000	2.660
120	.677	.845	1.041	1.289	1.658	1.980	2.617
∞	.674	.842	1.036	1.282	1.645	1.960	2.576

Source: W. J. Youden, *Statistical Methods for Chemists*. (New York and London: John Wiley & Sons, Inc., 1951.)
Text Explanation: pages 7, 13, 18, 23, 24.

Appendix Table 5

Tables for Testing Significance in 2×2 Tables with Unequal Samples

The table shows (1) in bold type for given a_1, n_1, and n_2, the value of a_2 which is just significant at the probability level quoted in parentheses (0.05) for a two-sided test and without parentheses for a one-sided test, (2) in small type, for given n_1, n_2, and $a_1 + a_2$, the exact probability (if there is independence) that a_2 is equal to or less than the integer shown in bold type.

Significance Level (left section)

n_1, n_2		a_1	0.05 (0.10)	0.025 (0.05)	0.01 (0.02)	0.005 (0.01)
$n_1=3$ $n_2=3$	3	3	0 .050	—	—	—
$n_1=4$ $n_2=4$	4	4	0 .014	0 .014	—	—
	3	4	0 .029	—	—	—
$n_1=5$ $n_2=5$	5	5	1 .024	1 .024	0 .004	0 .004
		4	0 .024	0 .024	—	—
	4	5	1 .048	0 .008	0 .008	—
		4	0 .040	—	—	—
	3	5	0 .018	0 .018	—	—
	2	5	0 .048	—	—	—
$n_1=6$ $n_2=6$	6	6	2 .030	1 .008	1 .008	0 .001
		5	1 .040	0 .008	0 .008	—
		4	0 .030	—	—	—
	5	6	1 .015+	1 .015+	0 .002	0 .002
		5	0 .013	0 .013	—	—
		4	0 .045+	—	—	—
	4	6	1 .033	0 .005-	0 .005-	0 .005-
		5	0 .024	—	—	—
	3	6	0 .012	0 .012	—	—
		5	0 .048	—	—	—
	2	6	0 .036	—	—	—
$n_1=7$ $n_2=7$	7	7	3 .035-	2 .010+	1 .002	1 .002
		6	1 .015-	1 .015-	0 .002	0 .002
		5	0 .010+	0 .010+	—	—
		4	0 .035-	—	—	—
	6	7	2 .021	2 .021	1 .005-	1 .005-
		6	1 .025+	0 .004	0 .004	0 .004
		5	0 .016	0 .016	—	—
		4	0 .049	—	—	—
	5	7	2 .045+	1 .010+	0 .001	0 .001
		6	1 .045+	0 .008	0 .008	—
		5	0 .027	—	—	—
	4	7	1 .024	1 .024	0 .003	0 .003
		6	0 .015+	0 .015+	—	—
		5	0 .045+	—	—	—
	3	7	0 .008	0 .008	0 .008	—
		6	0 .033	—	—	—
	2	7	0 .028	—	—	—

Significance Level (right section)

		a_1	0.05 (0.10)	0.025 (0.05)	0.01 (0.02)	0.005 (0.01)
$n_1=8$ $n_2=8$	8	8	4 .038	3 .013	2 .003	2 .003
		7	2 .020	2 .020	1 .005+	0 .001
		6	1 .020	1 .020	0 .003	0 .003
		5	0 .013	0 .013	—	—
		4	0 .038	—	—	—
	7	8	3 .026	2 .007	2 .007	1 .001
		7	2 .035-	1 .009	1 .009	0 .001
		6	1 .032	0 .006	0 .006	—
		5	0 .019	0 .019	—	—
	6	8	2 .015-	2 .015-	1 .003	1 .003
		7	1 .016	1 .016	0 .002	0 .002
		6	0 .009	0 .009	0 .009	—
		5	0 .028	—	—	—
	5	8	2 .035-	1 .007	1 .007	0 .001
		7	1 .032	0 .005-	0 .005-	0 .005-
		6	0 .016	0 .016	—	—
		5	0 .044	—	—	—
	4	8	1 .018	1 .018	0 .002	0 .002
		7	0 .010+	0 .010+	—	—
		6	0 .030	—	—	—
	3	8	0 .006	0 .006	0 .006	—
		7	0 .024	0 .024	—	—
	2	8	0 .022	0 .022	—	—
$n_1=9$ $n_2=9$	9	9	5 .041	4 .015-	3 .005-	3 .005-
		8	3 .025-	3 .025-	2 .008	1 .002
		7	2 .028	1 .008	1 .008	0 .001
		6	1 .025-	1 .025-	0 .005-	0 .005-
		5	0 .015-	0 .015-	—	—
		4	0 .041	—	—	—
	8	9	4 .029	3 .009	3 .009	2 .002
		8	3 .043	2 .013	1 .003	1 .003
		7	2 .044	1 .012	0 .002	0 .002
		6	1 .036	0 .007	0 .007	—
		5	0 .020	0 .020	—	—
	7	9	3 .019	3 .019	2 .005-	2 .005-
		8	2 .024	2 .024	1 .006	0 .001
		7	1 .020	1 .020	0 .003	0 .003
		6	0 .010+	0 .010+	—	—
		5	0 .029	—	—	—
	6	9	2 .044	2 .011	1 .002	1 .002
		8	2 .047	1 .011	0 .001	0 .001
		7	1 .035-	0 .006	0 .006	—
		6	0 .017	0 .017	—	—
		5	0 .042	—	—	—

Source: M. G. Natrella, *Experimental Statistics*. National Bureau of Standards Handbook 91 (Washington, D.C.: U.S. Government Printing Office, 1966, 1976).
Text Explanation: pages 29, 30.

Appendix Table 5 (Continued)
Tables for Testing Significance in 2 × 2 Tables with Unequal Samples

Left section

			Significance Level			
		a_1	0.05 (0.10)	0.025 (0.05)	0.01 (0.02)	0.005 (0.01)
$n_1=9$ $n_2=5$	9	9	2 .027	1 .005 −	1 .005 −	1 .005 −
		8	1 .023	1 .023	0 .003	0 .003
		7	0 .010 +	0 .010 +	—	—
		6	0 .028	—	—	—
	4	9	1 .014	1 .014	0 .001	0 .001
		8	0 .007	0 .007	0 .007	—
		7	0 .021	0 .021	—	—
		6	0 .049	—	—	—
	3	9	1 .045 +	0 .005 −	0 .005 −	0 .005 −
		8	0 .018	0 .018	—	—
		7	0 .045 +	—	—	—
	2	9	0 .018	0 .018	—	—
$n_1=10$ $n_2=10$	10	10	6 .043	5 .016	4 .005 +	3 .002
		9	4 .029	3 .010 −	3 .010 −	2 .003
		8	3 .035 −	2 .012	1 .003	1 .003
		7	2 .035 −	1 .010 −	1 .010 −	0 .002
		6	1 .029	0 .005 +	0 .005 +	—
		5	0 .016	0 .016	—	—
		4	0 .043	—	—	—
	9	10	5 .033	4 .011	3 .003	3 .003
		9	4 .050 −	3 .017	2 .005 −	2 .005 −
		8	2 .019	2 .019	1 .004	1 .004
		7	1 .015 −	1 .015 −	0 .002	0 .002
		6	1 .040	0 .008	0 .008	—
		5	0 .022	0 .022	—	—
	8	10	4 .023	4 .023	3 .007	2 .002
		9	3 .032	2 .009	2 .009	1 .002
		8	2 .031	1 .008	1 .008	0 .001
		7	1 .023	1 .023	0 .004	0 .004
		6	0 .011	0 .011	—	—
		5	0 .029	—	—	—
	7	10	3 .015 −	3 .015 −	2 .003	2 .003
		9	2 .018	2 .018	1 .004	1 .004
		8	1 .013	1 .013	0 .002	0 .002
		7	1 .036	0 .006	0 .006	—
		6	0 .017	0 .017	—	—
		5	0 .041	—	—	—
	6	10	3 .036	2 .008	2 .008	1 .001
		9	2 .036	1 .008	1 .008	0 .001
		8	1 .024	1 .024	0 .003	0 .003
		7	0 .010 +	0 .010 +	—	—
		6	0 .026	—	—	—
	5	10	2 .022	2 .022	1 .004	1 .004
		9	1 .017	1 .017	0 .002	0 .002
		8	1 .047	0 .007	0 .007	—
		7	0 .019	0 .019	—	—
		6	0 .042	—	—	—

Right section

			Significance Level			
		a_1	0.05 (0.10)	0.025 (0.05)	0.01 (0.02)	0.005 (0.01)
$n_1=10$ $n_2=4$	10	10	1 .011	1 .011	0 .001	0 .001
		9	1 .041	0 .005 −	0 .005 −	0 .005 −
		8	0 .015 −	0 .015 −	—	—
		7	0 .035 −	—	—	—
	3	10	1 .038	0 .003	0 .003	0 .003
		9	0 .014	0 .014	—	—
		8	0 .035 −	—	—	—
	2	10	0 .015 +	0 .015 +	—	—
		9	0 .045 +	—	—	—
$n_1=11$ $n_2=11$	11	11	7 .045 +	6 .018	5 .006	4 .002
		10	5 .032	4 .012	3 .004	3 .004
		9	4 .040	3 .015 −	2 .004	2 .004
		8	3 .043	2 .015 −	1 .004	1 .004
		7	2 .040	1 .012	0 .002	0 .002
		6	1 .032	0 .006	0 .006	—
		5	0 .018	0 .018	—	—
		4	0 .045 +	—	—	—
	10	11	6 .035 +	5 .012	4 .004	4 .004
		10	4 .021	4 .021	3 .007	2 .002
		9	3 .024	3 .024	2 .007	1 .002
		8	2 .023	2 .023	1 .006	0 .001
		7	1 .017	1 .017	0 .003	0 .003
		6	1 .043	0 .009	0 .009	—
		5	0 .023	0 .023	—	—
	9	11	5 .020	4 .008	4 .008	3 .002
		10	4 .038	3 .012	2 .003	2 .003
		9	3 .040	2 .012	1 .003	1 .003
		8	2 .035 −	1 .009	1 .009	0 .001
		7	1 .025 −	1 .025 −	0 .004	0 .004
		6	0 .012	0 .012	—	—
		5	0 .030	—	—	—
	8	11	4 .018	4 .018	3 .005 −	3 .005 −
		10	3 .024	3 .024	2 .006	1 .001
		9	2 .022	2 .022	1 .005 −	1 .005 −
		8	1 .015 −	1 .015 −	0 .002	0 .002
		7	1 .037	0 .007	0 .007	—
		6	0 .017	0 .017	—	—
		5	0 .040	—	—	—
	7	11	4 .043	3 .011	2 .002	2 .002
		10	3 .047	2 .013	1 .002	1 .002
		9	2 .039	1 .009	1 .009	0 .001
		8	1 .025 −	1 .025 −	0 .004	0 .004
		7	0 .010 +	0 .010 +	—	—
		6	0 .025 −	0 .025 −	—	—
	6	11	3 .029	2 .006	2 .006	1 .001
		10	2 .028	1 .005 +	1 .005 +	0 .001
		9	1 .018	1 .018	0 .002	0 .002

Left half

	a_1	Significance Level 0.05 (0.10)	0.025 (0.05)	0.01 (0.02)	0.005 (0.01)
$n_1=11$ $n_2=6$	8	1 .043	0 .007	0 .007	—
	7	0 .017	0 .017	—	—
	6	0 .037	—	—	—
5	11	2 .018	2 .018	1 .003	1 .003
	10	1 .013	1 .013	0 .001	0 .001
	9	1 .036	0 .005 −	0 .005 −	0 .005 −
	8	0 .013	0 .013	—	—
	7	0 .029	—	—	—
4	11	1 .009	1 .009	1 .009	0 .001
	10	1 .033	0 .004	0 .004	0 .004
	9	0 .011	0 .011	—	—
	8	0 .026	—	—	—
3	11	1 .033	0 .003	0 .003	0 .003
	10	0 .011	0 .011	—	—
	9	0 .027	—	—	—.
2	11	0 .013	0 .013	—	—
	10	0 .038	—	—	—
$n_1=12$ $n_2=12$	12	8 .047	7 .019	6 .007	5 .002
	11	6 .034	5 .014	4 .005 −	4 .005 −
	10	5 .045 −	4 .018	3 .006	2 .002
	9	4 .050 −	3 .020	2 .006	1 .001
	8	3 .050 −	2 .018	1 .005 −	1 .005 −
	7	2 .045 −	1 .014	0 .002	0 .002
	6	1 .034	0 .007	0 .007	—
	5	0 .019	0 .019	—	—
	4	0 .047	—	—	—
11	12	7 .037	6 .014	5 .005 −	5 .005 −
	11	5 .024	5 .024	4 .008	3 .002
	10	4 .029	3 .010 +	2 .003	2 .003
	9	3 .030	2 .009	2 .009	1 .002
	8	2 .026	1 .007	1 .007	0 .001
	7	1 .019	1 .019	0 .003	0 .003
	6	1 .045 −	0 .009	0 .009	—
	5	0 .024	0 .024	—	—
10	12	6 .029	5 .010 −	5 .010 −	4 .003
	11	5 .043	4 .015 +	3 .005 −	3 .005 −
	10	4 .048	3 .017	2 .005 −	2 .005 −
	9	3 .046	2 .015 −	1 .004	1 .004
	8	2 .038	1 .010 +	0 .002	0 .002
	7	1 .026	0 .005 −	0 .005 −	0 .005 −
	6	0 .012	0 .012	—	—
	5	0 .030	—	—	—
9	12	5 .021	5 .021	4 .006	3 .002
	11	4 .029	3 .009	3 .009	2 .002
	10	3 .029	2 .008	2 .008	1 .002
	9	2 .024	2 .024	1 .006	0 .001
	8	1 .016	1 .016	0 .002	0 .002

Right half

	a_1	Significance Level 0.05 (0.10)	0.025 (0.05)	0.01 (0.02)	0.005 (0.01)
$n_1=12$ $n_2=9$	7	1 .037	0 .007	0 .007	—
	6	0 .017	0 .017	—	—
	5	0 .039	—	—	—
8	12	5 .049	4 .014	3 .004	3 .004
	11	3 .018	3 .018	2 .004	*2 .004
	10	2 .015 +	2 .015 +	1 .003	1 .003
	9	2 .040	1 .010 −	1 .010 −	0 .001
	8	1 .025 −	1 .025 −	0 .004	0 .004
	7	0 .010 +	0 .010 +	—	—
	6	0 .024	0 .024	—	—
7	12	4 .036	3 .009	3 .009	2 .002
	11	3 .038	2 .010 −	2 .010 −	1 .002
	10	2 .029	1 .006	1 .006	0 .001
	9	1 .017	1 .017	0 .002	0 .002
	8	1 .040	0 .007	0 .007	—
	7	0 .016	0 .016	—	—
	6	0 .034	—	—	—
6	12	3 .025 −	3 .025 −	2 .005 −	2 .005 −
	11	2 .022	2 .022	1 .004	1 .004
	10	1 .013	1 .013	0 .002	0 .002
	9	1 .032	0 .005 −	0 .005 −	0 .005 −
	8	0 .011	0 .011	—	—
	7	0 .025 −	0 .025 −	—	—
	6	0 .050 −	—	—	—
5	12	2 .015 −	2 .015 −	1 .002	1 .002
	11	1 .010 −	1 .010 −	1 .010 −	0 .001
	10	1 .028	0 .003	0 .003	0 .003
	9	0 .009	0 .009	0 .009	—
	8	0 .020	0 .020	—	—
	7	0 .041	—	—	—
4	12	2 .050	1 .007	1 .007	0 .001
	11	1 .027	0 .003	0 .003	0 .003
	10	0 .008	0 .008	0 .008	—
	9	0 .019	0 .019	—	—
	8	0 .038	—	—	—
3	12	1 .029	0 .002	0 .002	0 .002
	11	0 .009	0 .009	0 .009	—
	10	0 .022	0 .022	—	—
	9	0 .044	—	—	—
2	12	0 .011	0 .011	—	—
	11	0 .033	—	—	—
$n_1=13$ $n_2=13$	13	9 .048	8 .020	7 .007	6 .003
	12	7 .037	6 .015 +	5 :006	4 .002
	11	6 .048	5 .021	4 .008	3 .002
	10	4 .024	4 .024	3 .008	2 .002
	9	3 .024	3 .024	2 .008	1 .002
	8	2 .021	2 .021	1 .006	0 .001

Appendix Table 5 (Continued)

Tables for Testing Significance in 2×2 Tables with Unequal Samples

Left block:

		a_1	0.05 (0.10)	0.025 (0.05)	0.01 (0.02)	0.005 (0.01)
$n_1=13$ $n_2=13$		7	2 .048	1 .015 +	0 .003	0 .003
		6	1 .037	0 .007	0 .007	—
		5	0 .020	0 .020	—	—
		4	0 .048	—	—	—
	12	13	8 .039	7 .015 −	6 .005 +	5 .002
		12	6 .027	5 .010 −	5 .010 −	4 .003
		11	5 .033	4 .013	3 .004	3 .004
		10	4 .036	3 .013	2 .004	2 .004
		9	3 .034	2 .011	1 .003	1 .003
		8	2 .029	1 .008	1 .008	0 .001
		7	1 .020	1 .020	0 .004	0 .004
		6	1 .046	0 .010 −	0 .010 −	—
		5	0 .024	0 .024	—	—
	11	13	7 .031	6 .011	5 .003	5 .003
		12	6 .048	5 .018	4 .006	3 .002
		11	4 .021	4 .021	3 .007	2 .002
		10	3 .021	3 .021	2 .006	1 .001
		9	3 .050 −	2 .017	1 .004	1 .004
		8	2 .040	1 .011	0 .002	0 .002
		7	1 .027	0 .005 −	0 .005 −	0 .005 −
		6	0 .013	0 .013	—	—
		5	0 .030	—	—	—
	10	13	6 .024	6 .024	5 .007	4 .002
		12	5 .035 −	4 .012	3 .003	3 .003
		11	4 .037	3 .012	2 .003	2 .003
		10	3 .033	2 .010 +	1 .002	1 .002
		9	2 .026	1 .006	1 .006	0 .001
		8	1 .017	1 .017	0 .003	0 .003
		7	1 .038	0 .007	0 .007	—
		6	0 .017	0 .017	—	—
		5	0 .038	—	—	—
	9	13	5 .017	5 .017	4 .005 −	4 .005 −
		12	4 .023	4 .023	3 .007	2 .001
		11	3 .022	3 .022	2 .006	1 .001
		10	2 .017	2 .017	1 .004	1 .004
		9	2 .040	1 .010 +	0 .001	0 .001
		8	1 .025 −	1 .025 −	0 .004	0 .004
		7	0 .010 +	0 .010 +	—	—
		6	0 .023	0 .023	—	—
		5	0 .049	—	—	—
	8	13	5 .042	4 .012	3 .003	3 .003
		12	4 .047	3 .014	2 .003	2 .003
		11	3 .041	2 .011	1 .002	1 .002
		10	2 .029	1 .007	1 .007	0 .001
		9	1 .017	1 .017	0 .002	0 .002
		8	1 .037	0 .006	0 .006	—
		7	0 .015 −	0 .015 −	—	—
		6	0 .032	—	—	—
	7	13	4 .031	3 .007	3 .007	2 .001
		12	3 .031	2 .007	2 .007	1 .001

Right block:

		a_1	0.05 (0.10)	0.025 (0.05)	0.01 (0.02)	0.005 (0.01)
$n_1=13$ $n_2=7$		11	2 .022	2 .022	1 .004	1 .004
		10	1 .012	1 .012	0 .002	0 .002
		9	1 .029	0 .004	0 .004	0 .004
		8	0 .010 +	0 .010 +	—	—
		7	0 .022	0 .022	—	—
		6	0 .044	—	—	—
	6	13	3 .021	3 .021	2 .004	2 .004
		12	2 .017	2 .017	1 .003	1 .003
		11	2 .046	1 .010 −	1 .010 −	0 .001
		10	1 .024	1 .024	0 .003	0 .003
		9	1 .050 −	0 .008	0 .008	—
		8	0 .017	0 .017	—	—
		7	0 .034	—	—	—
	5	13	2 .012	2 .012	1 .002	1 .002
		12	2 .044	1 .008	1 .008	0 .001
		11	1 .022	1 .022	0 .002	0 .022
		10	1 .047	0 .007	0 .007	—
		9	0 .015 −	0 .015 −	—	—
		8	0 .029	—	—	—
	4	13	2 .044	1 .006	1 .006	0 .000
		12	1 .022	1 .022	0 .002	0 .002
		11	0 .006	0 .006	0 .006	—
		10	0 .015 −	0 .015 −	—	—
		9	0 .029	—	—	—
	3	13	1 .025	1 .025	0 .002	0 .002
		12	0 .007	0 .007	0 .007	—
		11	0 .018	0 .018	—	—
		10	0 .036	—	—	—
	2	13	0 .010 −	0 .010 −	0 .010 −	—
		12	0 .029	—	—	—
$n_1=14$ $n_2=14$		14	10 .049	9 .020	8 .008	7 .003
		13	8 .038	7 .016	6 .006	5 .002
		12	6 .023	6 .023	5 .009	4 .002
		11	5 .027	4 .011	3 .004	3 .004
		10	4 .028	3 .011	2 .003	2 .003
		9	3 .027	2 .009	2 .009	1 .002
		8	2 .023	2 .023	1 .006	0 .001
		7	1 .016	1 .016	0 .003	0 .003
		6	1 .038	0 .008	0 .008	—
		5	0 .020	0 .020	—	—
		4	0 .049	—	—	—
	13	14	9 .041	8 .016	7 .006	6 .002
		13	7 .029	6 .011	5 .004	5 .004
		12	6 .037	5 .015 +	4 .005 +	3 .002
		11	5 .041	4 .017	3 .006	2 .001
		10	4 .041	3 .016	2 .005 −	2 .005 −
		9	3 .038	2 .013	1 .003	1 .003
		8	2 .031	1 .009	1 .009	0 .001

bles for Testing Significance in 2 × 2 Tables with Unequal Samples

			Significance Level							Significance Level			
		a_1	0.05 (0.10)	0.025 (0.05)	0.01 (0.02)	0.005 (0.01)			a_1	0.05 (0.10)	0.025 (0.05)	0.01 (0.02)	0.005 (0.01)
$n_1=14$ $n_2=13$		7	1 .021	1 .021	0 .004	0 .004	$n_1=14$ $n_2=7$		14	4 .026	3 .006	3 .006	2 .001
		6	1 .048	0 .010 +	—	—			13	3 .025	2 .006	2 .006	1 .001
		5	0 .025 −	0 .025 −	—	—			12	2 .017	2 .017	1 .003	1 .003
	12	14	8 .033	7 .012	6 .004	6 .004			11	2 .041	1 .009	1 .009	0 .001
		13	6 .021	6 .021	5 .007	4 .002			10	1 .021	1 .021	0 .003	0 .003
		12	5 .025 +	4 .009	4 .009	3 .003			9	1 .043	0 .007	0 .007	—
		11	4 .026	3 .009	3 .009	2 .002			8	0 .015 −	0 .015 −	—	—
		10	3 .024	3 .024	2 .007	1 .002			7	0 .030	—	—	—
		9	2 .019	2 .019	1 .005 −	1 .005 −		6	14	3 .018	3 .018	2 .003	2 .003
		8	2 .042	1 .012	0 .002	0 .002			13	2 .014	2 .014	1 .002	1 .002
		7	1 .028	0 .005 +	0 .005 +	—			12	2 .037	1 .007	1 .007	0 .001
		6	0 .013	0 .013	—	—			11	1 .018	1 .018	0 .002	0 .002
		5	0 .030	—	—	—			10	1 .038	0 .005 +	0 .005 +	—
	11	14	7 .026	6 .009	6 .009	5 .003			9	0 .012	0 .012	—	—
		13	6 .039	5 .014	4 .004	4 .004			8	0 .024	0 .024	—	—
		12	5 .043	4 .016	3 .005 −	3 .005 −			7	0 .044	—	—	—
		11	4 .042	3 .015 −	2 .004	2 .004		5	14	2 .010 +	2 .010 +	1 .001	1 .001
		10	3 .036	2 .011	1 .003	1 .003			13	2 .037	1 .006	1 .006	0 .001
		9	2 .027	1 .007	1 .007	0 .001			12	1 .017	1 .017	0 .002	0 .002
		8	1 .017	1 .017	0 .003	0 .003			11	1 .038	0 .005 −	0 .005 −	0 .005 −
		7	1 .038	0 .007	0 .007	—			10	0 .011	0 .011	—	—
		6	0 .017	0 .017	—	—			9	0 .022	0 .022	—	—
		5	0 .038	—	—	—			8	0 .040	—	—	—
	10	14	6 .020	6 .020	5 .006	4 .002		4	14	2 .039	1 .005 −	1 .005 −	1 .005 −
		13	5 .028	4 .009	4 .009	3 .002			13	1 .019	1 .019	0 .002	0 .002
		12	4 .028	3 .009	3 .009	2 .002			12	1 .044	0 .005 −	0 .005 −	0 .005 −
		11	3 .024	3 .024	2 .007	1 .001			11	0 .011	0 .011	—	—
		10	2 .018	2 .018	1 .004	1 .004			10	0 .023	0 .023	—	—
		9	2 .040	1 .011	0 .002	0 .002			9	0 .041	—	—	—
		8	1 .024	1 .024	0 .004	0 .004		3	14	1 .022	1 .022	0 .001	0 .001
		7	0 .010 −	0 .010 −	0 .010 −	—			13	0 .006	0 .006	0 .006	—
		6	0 .022	0 .022	—	—			12	0 .015 −	0 .015 −	—	—
		5	0 .047	—	—	—			11	0 .029	—	—	—
	9	14	6 .047	5 .014	4 .004	4 .004		2	14	0 .008	0 .008	0 .008	—
		13	4 .018	4 .018	3 .005 −	3 .005 −			13	0 .025	0 .025	—	—
		12	3 .017	3 .017	2 .004	2 .004			12	0 .050	—	—	—
		11	3 .042	2 .012	1 .002	1 .002	$n_1=15$ $n_2=15$		15	11 .050 −	10 .021	9 .008	8 .003
		10	2 .029	1 .007	1 .007	0 .001			14	9 .040	8 .018	7 .007	6 .003
		9	1 .017	1 .017	0 .002	0 .002			13	7 .025 +	6 .010 +	5 .004	5 .004
		8	1 .036	0 .006	0 .006	—			12	6 .030	5 .013	4 .005 −	4 .005 −
		7	0 .014	0 .014	—	—			11	5 .033	4 .013	3 .005 −	3 .005 −
		6	0 .030	—	—	—			10	4 .033	3 .013	2 .004	2 .004
	8	14	5 .036	4 .010 −	4 .010 −	3 .002			9	3 .030	2 .010 +	1 .003	1 .003
		13	4 .039	3 .011	2 .002	2 .002			8	2 .025 +	1 .007	1 .007	0 .001
		12	3 .032	2 .008	2 .008	1 .001			7	1 .018	1 .018	0 .003	0 .003
		11	2 .022	2 .022	1 .005 −	1 .005 −			6	1 .040	0 .008	0 .008	—
		10	2 .048	1 .012	0 .002	0 .002			5	0 .021	0 .021	—	—
		9	1 .026	0 .004	0 .004	0 .004			4	0 .050 −	—	—	—
		8	0 .009	0 .009	0 .009	—							
		7	0 .020	0 .020	—	—							
		6	0 .040	—	—	—							

Appendix Table 5 (Continued)
Tables for Testing Significance in 2 × 2 Tables with Unequal Samples

Left table — $n_1 = 15$, $n_2 = 14$

			Significance Level			
		a_1	0.05 (0.10)	0.025 (0.05)	0.01 (0.02)	0.005 (0.01)
$n_1=15$	$n_2=14$	15	10 .042	9 .017	8 .006	7 .002
		14	8 .031	7 .013	6 .005 −	6 .005 −
		13	7 .041	6 .017	5 .007	4 .002
		12	6 .046	5 .020	4 .007	3 .002
		11	5 .048	4 .020	3 .007	2 .002
		10	4 .046	3 .018	2 .006	1 .001
		9	3 .041	2 .014	1 .004	1 .004
		8	2 .033	1 .009	1 .009	0 .001
		7	1 .022	1 .022	0 .004	0 .004
		6	1 .049	0 .011	—	—
		5	0 .025 +	—	—	—
	13	15	9 .035 −	8 .013	7 .005 −	7 .005 −
		14	7 .023	7 .023	6 .009	5 .003
		13	6 .029	5 .011	4 .004	4 .004
		12	5 .031	4 .012	3 .004	3 .004
		11	4 .030	3 .011	2 .003	2 .003
		10	3 .026	2 .008	2 .008	1 .002
		9	2 .020	2 .020	1 .005 +	0 .001
		8	2 .043	1 .013	0 .002	0 .002
		7	1 .029	0 .005 +	0 .005 +	—
		6	0 .013	0 .013	—	—
		5	0 .031	—	—	—
	12	15	8 .028	7 .010 −	7 .010 −	6 .003
		14	7 .043	6 .016	5 .006	4 .002
		13	6 .049	5 .019	4 .007	3 .002
		12	5 .049	4 .019	3 .006	2 .002
		11	4 .045 +	3 .017	2 .005 −	2 .005 −
		10	3 .038	2 .012	1 .003	1 .003
		9	2 .028	1 .007	1 .007	0 .001
		8	1 .018	1 .018	0 .003	0 .003
		7	1 .038	0 .007	0 .007	—
		6	0 .017	0 .017	—	—
		5	0 .037	—	—	—
	11	15	7 .022	7 .022	6 .007	5 .002
		14	6 .032	5 .011	4 .003	4 .003
		13	5 .034	4 .012	3 .003	3 .003
		12	4 .032	3 .010 +	2 .003	2 .003
		11	3 .026	2 .008	2 .008	1 .002
		10	2 .019	2 .019	1 .004	1 .004
		9	2 .040	1 .011	0 .002	0 .002
		8	1 .024	1 .024	0 .004	0 .004
		7	1 .049	0 .010 −	0 .010 −	—
		6	0 .022	0 .022	—	—
		5	0 .046	—	—	—
	10	15	6 .017	6 .017	5 .005 −	5 .005 −
		14	5 .023	5 .023	4 .007	3 .002
		13	4 .022	4 .022	3 .007	2 .001
		12	3 .018	3 .018	2 .005 −	2 .005 −
		11	3 .042	2 .013	1 .003	1 .003
		10	2 .029	1 .007	1 .007	0 .001
		9	1 .016	1 .016	0 .002	0 .002
		8	1 .034	0 .006	0 .006	—
		7	0 .013	0 .013	—	—
		6	0 .028	—	—	—
	9	15	6 .042	5 .012	4 .003	4 .003
		14	5 .047	4 .015 −	3 .004	3 .004

Right table — $n_1 = 15$, $n_2 = 9$

			Significance Level			
		a_1	0.05 (0.10)	0.025 (0.05)	0.01 (0.02)	0.005 (0.01)
$n_1=15$	$n_2=9$	13	4 .042	3 .013	2 .003	2 .003
		12	3 .032	2 .009	2 .009	1 .002
		11	2 .021	2 .021	1 .005 −	1 .005
		10	2 .045 −	1 .011	0 .002	0 .002
		9	1 .024	1 .024	0 .004	0 .004
		8	1 .048	0 .009	0 .009	—
		7	0 .019	0 .019	—	—
		6	0 .037	—	—	—
	8	15	5 .032	4 .008	4 .008	3 .002
		14	4 .033	3 .009	3 .009	2 .002
		13	3 .026	2 .006	2 .006	1 .001
		12	2 .017	2 .017	1 .003	1 .003
		11	2 .037	1 .008	1 .008	0 .001
		10	1 .019	1 .019	0 .003	0 .003
		9	1 .038	0 .006	0 .006	—
		8	0 .013	0 .013	—	—
		7	0 .026	—	—	—
		6	0 .050 −	—	—	—
	7	15	4 .023	4 .023	3 .005 −	3 .005
		14	3 .021	3 .021	2 .004	2 .004
		13	2 .014	2 .014	1 .002	1 .002
		12	2 .032	1 .007	1 .007	0 .001
		11	1 .015 +	1 .015 +	0 .002	0 .002
		10	1 .032	0 .005 −	0 .005 −	0 .005
		9	0 .010 +	0 .010 +	—	—
		8	0 .020	0 .020	—	—
		7	0 .038	—	—	—
	6	15	3 .015 +	3 .015 +	2 .003	2 .003
		14	2 .011	2 .011	1 .002	1 .002
		13	2 .031	1 .006	1 .006	0 .001
		12	1 .014	1 .014	0 .002	0 .002
		11	1 .029	0 .004	0 .004	0 .004
		10	0 .009	0 .009	0 .009	—
		9	0 .017	0 .017	—	—
		8	0 .032	—	—	—
	5	15	2 .009	2 .009	2 .009	1 .001
		14	2 .032	1 .005 −	1 .005 −	1 .005
		13	1 .014	1 .014	0 .001	0 .001
		12	1 .031	0 .004	0 .004	0 .004
		11	0 .008	0 .008	0 .008	—
		10	0 .016	0 .016	—	—
		9	0 .030	—	—	—
	4	15	2 .035 +	1 .004	1 .004	1 .004
		14	1 .016	1 .016	0 .001	0 .001
		13	1 .037	0 .004	0 .004	0 .004
		12	0 .009	0 .009	0 .009	—
		11	0 .018	0 .018	—	—
		10	0 .033	—	—	—
	3	15	1 .020	1 .020	0 .001	0 .001
		14	0 .005 −	0 .005 −	0 .005 −	0 .005 −
		13	0 .012	0 .012	—	—
		12	0 .025 −	0 .025 −	—	—
		11	0 .043	—	—	—
	2	15	0 .007	0 .007	0 .007	—
		14	0 .022	0 .022	—	—
		13	0 .044	—	—	—

$n_1 = 16$, $n_2 = 16$

	a_1	0.05 (0.10)	0.025 (0.05)	0.01 (0.02)	0.005 (0.01)
16	16	11 .022	11 .022	10 .009	9 .003
	15	10 .041	9 .019	8 .008	7 .003
	14	8 .027	7 .012	6 .005 −	6 .005 −
	13	7 .033	6 .015 −	5 .006	4 .002
	12	6 .037	5 .016	4 .006	3 .002
	11	5 .038	4 .016	3 .006	2 .002
	10	4 .037	3 .015 −	2 .005 −	2 .005 −
	9	3 .033	2 .012	1 .003	1 .003
	8	2 .027	1 .008	1 .008	0 .001
	7	1 .019	1 .019	0 .003	0 .003
	6	1 .041	0 .009	0 .009	—
	5	0 .022	0 .022	—	—
15	16	11 .043	10 .018	9 .007	8 .002
	15	9 .033	8 .014	7 .005 +	6 .002
	14	8 .044	7 .019	6 .008	5 .003
	13	6 .023	6 .023	5 .009	4 .003
	12	5 .024	5 .024	4 .009	3 .003
	11	4 .023	4 .023	3 .008	2 .002
	10	4 .049	3 .020	2 .006	1 .001
	9	3 .043	2 .016	1 .004	1 .004
	8	2 .035 −	1 .010 +	0 .002	0 .002
	7	1 .023	1 .023	0 .004	0 .004
	6	0 .011	0 .011	—	—
	5	0 .026	—	—	—
14	16	10 .037	9 .014	8 .005 +	7 .002
	15	8 .025 +	7 .010 −	7 .010 −	6 .003
	14	7 .032	6 .013	5 .005 −	5 .005 −
	13	6 .035 +	5 .014	4 .005 +	3 .001
	12	5 .035 +	4 .014	3 .005 −	3 .005 −
	11	4 .033	3 .012	2 .004	2 .004
	10	3 .028	2 .009	2 .009	1 .002
	9	2 .021	2 .021	1 .006	0 .001
	8	2 .045 −	1 .013	0 .002	0 .002
	7	1 .030	0 .006	0 .006	—
	6	0 .013	0 .013	—	—
	5	0 .031	—	—	—
13	16	9 .030	8 .011	7 .004	7 .004
	15	8 .047	7 .019	6 .007	5 .002
	14	6 .023	6 .023	5 .008	4 .003
	13	5 .023	5 .023	4 .008	3 .003
	12	4 .022	4 .022	3 .007	2 .002
	11	4 .048	3 .018	2 .005 +	1 .001
	10	3 .039	2 .013	1 .003	1 .003
	9	2 .029	1 .008	1 .008	0 .001
	8	1 .018	1 .018	0 .003	0 .003
	7	1 .038	0 .007	0 .007	—
	6	0 .017	0 .017	—	—
	5	0 .037	—	—	—

$n_1 = 16$, $n_2 = 12$

	a_1	0.05 (0.10)	0.025 (0.05)	0.01 (0.02)	0.005 (0.01)
16	16	8 .024	8 .024	7 .008	6 .002
	15	7 .036	6 .013	5 .004	5 .004
	14	6 .040	5 .015 −	4 .005 −	4 .005 −
	13	5 .039	4 .014	3 .004	3 .004
	12	4 .034	3 .012	2 .003	2 .003
	11	3 .027	2 .008	2 .008	1 .002
	10	2 .019	2 .019	1 .005 −	1 .005 −
	9	2 .040	1 .011	0 .002	0 .002
	8	1 .024	1 .024	0 .004	0 .004
	7	1 .048	0 .010 −	0 .010 −	—
	6	0 .021	0 .021	—	—
	5	0 .044	—	—	—
11	16	7 .019	7 .019	6 .006	5 .002
	15	6 .027	5 .009	5 .009	4 .002
	14	5 .027	4 .009	4 .009	3 .002
	13	4 .024	4 .024	3 .008	2 .002
	12	3 .019	3 .019	2 .005 +	1 .001
	11	3 .041	2 .013	1 .003	1 .003
	10	2 .028	1 .007	1 .007	0 .001
	9	1 .016	1 .016	0 .002	0 .002
	8	1 .033	0 .006	0 .006	—
	7	0 .013	0 .013	—	—
	6	0 .027	—	—	—
10	16	7 .046	6 .014	5 .004	5 .004
	15	5 .018	5 .018	4 .005 +	3 .001
	14	4 .017	4 .017	3 .005 −	3 .005 −
	13	4 .042	3 .014	2 .003	2 .003
	12	3 .032	2 .009	2 .009	1 .002
	11	2 .021	2 .021	1 .005 −	1 .005 −
	10	2 .042	1 .011	0 .002	0 .002
	9	1 .023	1 .023	0 .004	0 .004
	8	1 .045 −	0 .008	0 .008	—
	7	0 .017	0 .017	—	—
	6	0 .035 −	—	—	—
9	16	6 .037	5 .010 −	5 .010 −	4 .002
	15	5 .040	4 .012	3 .003	3 .003
	14	4 .034	3 .010 −	3 .010 −	2 .002
	13	3 .025 +	2 .007	2 .007	1 .001
	12	2 .016	2 .016	1 .003	1 .003
	11	2 .033	1 .008	1 .008	0 .001
	10	1 .017	1 .017	0 .002	0 .002
	9	1 .034	0 .006	0 .006	—
	8	0 .012	0 .012	—	—
	7	0 .024	0 .024	—	—
	6	0 .045 +	—	—	—

Appendix Table 5 (Continued)
Tables for Testing Significance in 2 × 2 Tables with Unequal Samples

$n_1 = 16$, $n_2 = 8$

	a_1	Significance Level 0.05 (0.10)	0.025 (0.05)	0.01 (0.02)	0.005 (0.01)
$n_1=16$ $n_2=8$	16	5 .028	4 .007	4 .007	3 .001
	15	4 .028	3 .007	3 .007	2 .001
	14	3 .021	3 .021	2 .005 −	2 .005 −
	13	3 .047	2 .013	1 .002	1 .002
	12	2 .028	1 .006	1 .006	0 .001
	11	1 .014	1 .014	0 .002	0 .002
	10	1 .027	0 .004	0 .004	0 .004
	9	0 .009	0 .009	0 .009	—
	8	0 .017	0 .017	—	—
	7	0 .033	—	—	—
7	16	4 .020	4 .020	3 .004	3 .004
	15	3 .017	3 .017	2 .003	2 .003
	14	3 .045 +	2 .011	1 .002	1 .002
	13	2 .026	1 .005 −	1 .005 −	1 .005 −
	12	1 .012	1 .012	0 .001	0 .001
	11	1 .024	1 .024	0 .003	0 .003
	10	1 .045 −	0 .007	0 .007	—
	9	0 .014	0 .014	—	—
	8	0 .026	—	--	—
	7	0 .047	—	—	—
6	16	3 .013	3 .013	2 .002	2 .002
	15	3 .046	2 .009	2 .009	1 .001
	14	2 .025 +	1 .004	1 .004	1 .004
	13	1 .011	1 .011	0 .001	0 .001
	12	1 .023	1 .023	0 .003	0 .003
	11	1 .043	0 .006	0 .006	—
	10	0 .012	0 .012	—	—
	9	0 .023	0 .023	—	—
	8	0 .040	—	—	—
5	16	3 .048	2 .008	2 .008	1 .001
	15	2 .028	1 .004	1 .004	1 .004
	14	1 .011	1 .011	0 .001	0 .001
	13	1 .025 +	0 .003	0 .003	0 .003
	12	1 .047	0 .006	0 .006	—
	11	0 .012	0 .012	—	—
	10	0 .023	0 .023	—	—
	9	0 .039	—	—	—
4	16	2 .032	1 .004	1 .004	1 .004
	15	2 .013	1 .013	0 .001	0 .001
	14	1 .032	0 .003	0 .003	0 .003
	13	0 .007	0 .007	0 .007	—
	12	0 .014	0 .014	—	—
	11	0 .026	—	—	—
	10	0 .043	—	—	—

Right section

	a_1	Significance Level 0.05 (0.10)	0.025 (0.05)	0.01 (0.02)	0.005 (0.01)
$n_1=16$ $n_2=3$	16	1 .018	1 .018	0 .001	0 .001
	15	0 .004	0 .004	0 .004	0 .004
	14	0 .010 +	0 .010 +	—	—
	13	0 .021	0 .021	—	—
	12	0 .036	—	—	—
2	16	0 .007	0 .007	0 .007	—
	15	0 .020	0 .020	—	—
	14	0 .039	—	—	—
$n_1=17$ $n_2=17$	17	12 .022	12 .022	11 .009	10 .004
	16	11 .043	10 .020	9 .008	8 .003
	15	9 .029	8 .013	7 .005 +	6 .002
	14	8 .035 +	7 .016	6 .007	5 .002
	13	7 .040	6 .018	5 .007	4 .003
	12	6 .042	5 .019	4 .007	3 .002
	11	5 .042	4 .018	3 .007	2 .002
	10	4 .040	3 .016	2 .005 +	1 .001
	9	3 .035 +	2 .013	1 .003	1 .003
	8	2 .029	1 .008	1 .008	0 .001
	7	1 .020	1 .020	0 .004	0 .004
	6	1 .043	0 .009	0 .009	—
	5	0 .022	0 .022	—	—
16	17	12 .044	11 .018	10 .007	9 .003
	16	10 .035 −	9 .015 −	8 .006	7 .002
	15	9 .046	8 .021	7 .009	6 .003
	14	7 .025 +	6 .011	5 .004	5 .004
	13	6 .027	5 .011	4 .004	4 .004
	12	5 .027	4 .011	3 .004	3 .004
	11	4 .025 +	3 .009	3 .009	2 .003
	10	3 .022	3 .022	2 .007	1 .002
	9	3 .046	2 .017	1 .004	1 .004
	8	2 .036	1 .011	0 .002	0 .002
	7	1 .024	1 .024	0 .005 −	0 .005 −
	6	0 .011	0 .011	—	—
	5	0 .026	—	—	—
15	17	11 .038	10 .015 −	9 .006	8 .002
	16	9 .027	8 .011	7 .004	7 .004
	15	8 .035 +	7 .015 −	6 .006	5 .002
	14	7 .040	6 .017	5 .006	4 .002
	13	6 .041	5 .017	4 .006	3 .002
	12	5 .039	4 .016	3 .005 +	2 .001
	11	4 .035 +	3 .013	2 .004	2 .004
	10	3 .029	2 .010 −	2 .010 −	1 .002
	9	2 .022	2 .022	1 .006	0 .001
	8	2 .046	1 .014	0 .002	0 .002
	7	1 .030	0 .006	0 .006	—
	6	0 .014	0 .014	—	—
	5	0 .031	—	—	—

$n_1 = 17$ $n_2 = 14$

	a_1	Significance Level			
		0.05 (0.10)	0.025 (0.05)	0.01 (0.02)	0.005 (0.01)
	17	10 .032	9 .012	8 .004	8 .004
	16	8 .021	8 .021	7 .008	6 .003
	15	7 .026	6 .010 −	6 .010 −	5 .003
	14	6 .028	5 .011	4 .004	4 .004
	13	5 .027	4 .010 −	4 .010 −	3 .003
	12	4 .024	4 .024	3 .008	2 .002
	11	4 .049	3 .019	2 .006	1 .001
	10	3 .040	2 .014	1 .003	1 .003
	9	2 .029	1 .008	1 .008	0 .001
	8	1 .018	1 .018	0 .003	0 .003
	7	1 .038	0 .007	0 .007	—
	6	0 .017	0 .017	—	—
	5	0 .036	—	—	—
13	17	9 .026	8 .009	8 .009	7 .003
	16	8 .040	7 .015 +	6 .005 +	5 .002
	15	7 .045 +	6 .018	5 .006	4 .002
	14	6 .045 +	5 .018	4 .006	3 .002
	13	5 .042	4 .016	3 .005 +	2 .001
	12	4 .035 +	3 .013	2 .004	2 .004
	11	3 .028	2 .009	2 .009	1 .002
	10	2 .019	2 .019	1 .005 −	1 .005 −
	9	2 .040	1 .011	0 .002	0 .002
	8	1 .024	1 .024	0 .004	0 .004
	7	1 .047	0 .010 −	0 .010 −	—
	6	0 .021	0 .021	—	—
	5	0 .043	—	—	—
12	17	8 .021	8 .021	7 .007	6 .002
	16	7 .030	6 .011	5 .003	5 .003
	15	6 .033	5 .012	4 .004	4 .004
	14	5 .030	4 .011	3 .003	3 .003
	13	4 .026	3 .008	3 .008	2 .002
	12	3 .020	3 .020	2 .006	1 .001
	11	3 .041	2 .013	1 .003	1 .003
	10	2 .028	1 .007	1 .007	0 .001
	9	1 .016	1 .016	0 .002	0 .002
	8	1 .032	0 .006	0 .006	—
	7	0 .012	0 .012	—	—
	6	0 .026	—	—	—
11	17	7 .016	7 .016	6 .005 −	6 .005 −
	16	6 .022	6 .022	5 .007	4 .002
	15	5 .022	5 .022	4 .007	3 .002
	14	4 .019	4 .019	3 .006	2 .001

$n_1 = 17$ $n_2 = 11$

	a_1	Significance Level			
		0.05 (0.10)	0.025 (0.05)	0.01 (0.02)	0.005 (0.01)
	13	4 .042	3 .014	2 .004	2 .004
	12	3 .031	2 .009	2 .009	1 .002
	11	2 .020	2 .020	1 .005 −	1 .005 −
	10	2 .040	1 .011	0 .001	0 .001
	9	1 .022	1 .022	0 .004	0 .004
	8	1 .042	0 .008	0 .008	—
	7	0 .016	0 .016	—	—
	6	0 .033	—	—	—
10	17	7 .041	6 .012	5 .003	5 .003
	16	6 .047	5 .015 +	4 .004	4 .004
	15	5 .043	4 .014	3 .004	3 .004
	14	4 .034	3 .010 +	2 .002	2 .002
	13	3 .024	3 .024	2 .007	1 .001
	12	3 .049	2 .015 +	1 .003	1 .003
	11	2 .031	1 .007	1 .007	0 .001
	10	1 .016	1 .016	0 .002	0 .002
	9	1 .031	0 .005 +	0 .005 +	—
	8	0 .011	0 .011	—	—
	7	0 .022	0 .022	—	—
	6	0 .042	—	—	—
9	17	6 .032	5 .008	5 .008	4 .002
	16	5 .034	4 .010 −	4 .010 −	3 .002
	15	4 .028	3 .008	3 .008	2 .002
	14	3 .020	3 .020	2 .005 −	2 .005 −
	13	3 .042	2 .012	1 .002	1 .002
	12	2 .025 +	1 .006	1 .006	0 .001
	11	2 .048	1 .012	0 .002	0 .002
	10	1 .024	1 .024	0 .004	0 .004
	9	1 .045 −	0 .008	0 .008	—
	8	0 .016	0 .016	—	—
	7	0 .030	—	—	—
8	17	5 .024	5 .024	4 .006	3 .001
	16	4 .023	4 .023	3 .006	2 .001
	15	3 .017	3 .017	2 .004	2 .004
	14	3 .039	2 .010 −	2 .010 −	1 .002
	13	2 .022	2 .022	1 .004	1 .004
	12	2 .043	1 .010 −	1 .010 −	0 .001
	11	1 .020	1 .020	0 .003	0 .003
	10	1 .038	0 .006	0 .006	—
	9	0 .012	0 .012	—	—
	8	0 .022	0 .022	—	—
	7	0 .040	—	—	—

Appendix Table 5 (Continued)
Tables for Testing Significance in 2 × 2 Tables with Unequal Samples

			Significance Level							Significance Level			
		a_1	0.05 (0.10)	0.025 (0.05)	0.01 (0.02)	0.005 (0.01)			a_1	0.05 (0.10)	0.025 (0.05)	0.01 (0.02)	0.005 (0.01)
$n_1=17$ $n_2=7$		17	4 .017	4 .017	3 .003	3 .003	$n_1=18$ $n_2=18$		18	13 .023	13 .023	12 .010 −	11 .004
		16	3 .014	3 .014	2 .003	2 .003			17	12 .044	11 .020	10 .009	9 .004
		15	3 .038	2 .009	2 .009	1 .001			16	10 .030	9 .014	8 .006	7 .002
		14	2 .021	2 .021	1 .004	1 .004			15	9 .038	8 .018	7 .008	6 .003
		13	2 .042	1 .009	1 .009	0 .001			14	8 .043	7 .020	6 .009	5 .003
		12	1 .018	1 .018	0 .002	0 .002			13	7 .046	6 .022	5 .009	4 .003
		11	1 .034	0 .005 −	0 .005 −	0 .005 −			12	6 .047	5 .022	4 .009	3 .003
		10	0 .010 −	0 .010 −	0 .010 −	—			11	5 .046	4 .020	3 .008	2 .002
		9	0 .019	0 .019	—	—			10	4 .043	3 .018	2 .006	1 .001
		8	0 .033	—	—	—			9	3 .038	2 .014	1 .004	1 .004
	6	17	3 .011	3 .011	2 .002	2 .002			8	2 .030	1 .009	1 .009	0 .001
		16	3 .040	2 .008	2 .008	1 .001			7	1 .020	1 .020	0 .004	0 .004
		15	2 .021	2 .021	1 .003	1 .003			6	1 .044	0 .010 −	0 .010 −	—
		14	2 .045 +	1 .009	1 .009	1 .001			5	0 .023	0 .023 •	—	—
		13	1 .018	1 .018	0 .002	0 .002		17	18	13 .045 +	12 .019	11 .008	10 .003
		12	1 .035 −	0 .005 −	0 .005 −	0 .005 −			17	11 .036	10 .016	9 .007	8 .002
		11	0 .009	0 .009	0 .009	—			16	10 .049	9 .023	8 .010 −	7 .004
		10	0 .017	0 .017	—	—			15	8 .028	7 .012	6 .005 −	6 .005 −
		9	0 .030	—	—	—			14	7 .030	6 .013	5 .005 +	4 .002
		8	0 .050 −	—	—	—			13	6 .031	5 .013	4 .005 −	4 .005 −
	5	17	3 .043	2 .006	2 .006	1 .001			12	5 .030	4 .012	3 .004	3 .004
		16	2 .024	2 .024	1 .003	1 .003			11	4 .028	3 .010 +	2 .003	2 .003
		15	1 .009	1 .009	1 .009	0 .001			10	3 .023	3 .023	2 .008	1 .002
		14	1 .021	1 .021	0 .002	0 .002			9	3 .047	2 .018	1 .005 −	1 .005 −
		13	1 .039	0 .005 −	0 .005 −	0 .005 −			8	2 .037	1 .011	0 .002	0 .002
		12	0 .010 −	0 .010 −	0 .010 −	—			7	1 .025 −	1 .025 −	0 .005 −	0 .005 −
		11	0 .018	0 .018	—	—			6	0 .011	0 .011	—	—
		10	0 .030	—	—	—			5	0 .026	—	—	—
		9	0 .049	—	—	—		16	18	12 .039	11 .016	10 .006	9 .002
	4	17	2 .029	1 .003	1 .003	1 .003			17	10 .029	9 .012	8 .005 −	8 .005 −
		16	1 .012	1 .012	0 .001	0 .001			16	9 .038	8 .017	7 .007	6 .002
		15	1 .028	0 .003	0 .003	0 .003			15	8 .043	7 .019	6 .008	5 .003
		14	0 .006	0 .006	0 .006	—			14	7 .046	6 .020	5 .008	4 .003
		13	0 .012	0 .012	—	—			13	6 .045 +	5 .020	4 .007	3 .002
		12	0 .021	0 .021	—	—			12	5 .042	4 .018	3 .006	2 .002
		11	0 .035 +	—	—	—			11	4 .037	3 .015 −	2 .004	2 .004
	3	17	1 .016	1 .016	0 .001	0 .001			10	3 .031	2 .011	1 .003	1 .003
		16	1 .046	0 .004	0 .004	0 .004			9	2 .023	2 .023	1 .006	0 .001
		15	0 .009	0 .009	0 .009	—			8	2 .046	1 .014	0 .002	0 .002
		14	0 .018	0 .018	—	—			7	1 .030	0 .006	0 .006	—
		13	0 .031	—	—	—			6	0 .014	0 .014	—	—
		12	0 .049	—	—	—			5	0 .031	—	—	—
	2	17	0 .006	0 .006	0 .006	—		15	18	11 .033	10 .013	9 .005 −	9 .005 −
		16	0 .018	0 .018	—	—			17	9 .023	9 .023	8 .009	7 .003
		15	0 .035 +	—	—	—			16	8 .029	7 .012	6 .004	6 .004
									15	7 .031	6 .013	5 .005 −	5 .005 −
									14	6 .031	5 .013	4 .004	4 .004
									13	5 .029	4 .011	3 .004	3 .004

$n_1 = 18$ $n_2 = 15$

	a_1	0.05 (0.10)	0.025 (0.05)	0.01 (0.02)	0.005 (0.01)
15	12	4 .025+	3 .009	3 .009	2 .003
	11	3 .020	3 .020	2 .006	1 .001
	10	3 .041	2 .014	1 .004	1 .004
	9	2 .030	1 .008	1 .008	0 .001
	8	1 .018	1 .018	0 .003	0 .003
	7	1 .038	0 .007	0 .007	—
	6	0 .017	0 .017	—	—
	5	0 .036	—	—	—
14	18	10 .028	9 .010−	9 .010−	8 .003
	17	9 .043	8 .017	7 .006	6 .002
	16	8 .050−	7 .021	6 .008	5 .003
	15	6 .022	6 .022	5 .008	4 .003
	14	6 .049	5 .020	4 .007	3 .002
	13	5 .044	4 .017	3 .006	2 .001
	12	4 .037	3 .013	2 .004	2 .004
	11	3 .028	2 .009	2 .009	1 .002
	10	2 .020	2 .020	1 .005−	1 .005−
	9	2 .039	1 .011	0 .002	0 .002
	8	1 .024	1 .024	0 .004	0 .004
	7	1 .047	0 .009	0 .009	—
	6	0 .020	0 .020	—	—
	5	0 .043	—	—	—
13	18	9 .023	9 .023	8 .008	7 .002
	17	8 .034	7 .012	6 .004	6 .004
	16	7 .037	6 .014	5 .005−	5 .005−
	15	6 .036	5 .014	4 .004	4 .004
	14	5 .032	4 .012	3 .004	3 .004
	13	4 .027	3 .009	3 .009	2 .002
	12	3 .020	3 .020	2 .006	1 .001
	11	3 .040	2 .013	1 .003	1 .003
	10	2 .027	1 .007	1 .007	0 .001
	9	1 .015+	1 .015+	0 .002	0 .002
	8	1 .031	0 .006	0 .006	—
	7	0 .012	0 .012	—	—
	6	0 .025+	—	—	—
12	18	8 .018	8 .018	7 .006	6 .002
	17	7 .026	6 .009	6 .009	5 .003
	16	6 .027	5 .009	5 .009	4 .003
	15	5 .024	5 .024	4 .008	3 .002
	14	4 .020	4 .020	3 .006	2 .001
	13	4 .042	3 .014	2 .004	2 .004
	12	3 .030	2 .009	2 .009	1 .002
	11	2 .019	2 .019	1 .005−	1 .005−

$n_1 = 18$ $n_2 = 12$

	a_1	0.05 (0.10)	0.025 (0.05)	0.01 (0.02)	0.005 (0.01)
	10	2 .038	1 .010+	0 .001	0 .001
	9	1 .021	1 .021	0 .003	0 .003
	8	1 .040	0 .007	0 .007	—
	7	0 .016	0 .016	—	—
	6	0 .031	—	—	—
11	18	8 .045+	7 .014	6 .004	6 .004
	17	6 .018	6 .018	5 .006	4 .001
	16	5 .018	5 .018	4 .005+	3 .001
	15	5 .043	4 .015−	3 .004	3 .004
	14	4 .033	3 .011	2 .003	2 .003
	13	3 .023	3 .023	2 .007	1 .001
	12	3 .046	2 .014	1 .003	1 .003
	11	2 .029	1 .007	1 .007	0 .001
	10	1 .015−	1 .015−	0 .002	0 .002
	9	1 .029	0 .005−	0 .005−	0 .005−
	8	0 .010+	0 .010+	—	—
	7	0 .020	0 .020	—	—
	6	0 .039	—	—	—
10	18	7 .037	6 .010+	5 .003	5 .003
	17	6 .041	5 .013	4 .003	4 .003
	16	5 .036	4 .011	3 .003	3 .003
	15	4 .028	3 .008	3 .008	2 .002
	14	3 .019	3 .019	2 .005−	2 .005−
	13	3 .039	2 .011	1 .002	1 .002
	12	2 .023	2 .023	1 .005+	0 .001
	11	2 .043	1 .011	0 .001	0 .001
	10	1 .022	1 .022	0 .003	0 .003
	9	1 .040	0 .007	0 .007	—
	8	0 .014	0 .014	—	—
	7	0 .027	—	—	—
	6	0 .049	—	—.	—
9	18	6 .029	5 .007	5 .007	4 .002
	17	5 .030	4 .008	4 .008	3 .002
	16	4 .023	4 .023	3 .006	2 .001
	15	3 .016	3 .016	2 .004	2 .004
	14	3 .034	2 .009	2 .009	1 .002
	13	2 .019	2 .019	1 .004	1 .004
	12	2 .037	1 .009	1 .009	0 .001
	11	1 .018	1 .018	0 .002	0 .002
	10	1 .033	0 .005+	0 .005+	—
	9	0 .010+	0 .010+	—	—
	8	0 .020	0 .020	—	—
	7	0 .036	—	—	—

Tables for Testing Significance in 2 × 2 Tables with Unequal Samples

		a_1	Significance Level 0.05 (0.10)	0.025 (0.05)	0.01 (0.02)	0.005 (0.01)
$n_1=18$ $n_2=8$		18	5 .022	5 .022	4 .005−	4 .005−
		17	4 .020	4 .020	3 .004	3 .004
		16	3 .014	3 .014	2 .003	2 .003
		15	3 .032	2 .008	2 .008	1 .001
		14	2 .017	2 .017	1 .003	1 .003
		13	2 .034	1 .007	1 .007	0 .001
		12	1 .015+	1 .015+	0 .002	0 .002
		11	1 .028	0 .004	0 .004	0 .004
		10	1 .049	0 .008	0 .008	—
		9	0 .016	0 .016	—	—
		8	0 .028	—	—	—
		7	0 .048	—	—	—
	7	18	4 .015+	4 .015+	3 .003	3 .003
		17	3 .012	3 .012	2 .002	2 .002
		16	3 .032	2 .007	2 .007	1 .001
		15	2 .017	2 .017	1 .003	1 .003
		14	2 .034	1 .007	1 .007	0 .001
		13	1 .014	1 .014	0 .002	0 .002
		12	1 .027	0 .004	0 .004	0 .004
		11	1 .046	0 .007	0 .007	—
		10	0 .013	0 .013	—	—
		9	0 .024	0 .024	—	—
		8	0 .040	—	—	—
	6	18	3 .010−	3 .010−	3 .010−	2 .001
		17	3 .035+	2 .006	2 .006	1 .001
		16	2 .018	2 .018	1 .003	1 .003
		15	2 .038	1 .007	1 .007	0 .001
		14	1 .015−	1 .015−	0 .002	0 .002
		13	1 .028	0 .003	0 .003	0 .003
		12	1 .048	0 .007	0 .007	—
		11	0 .013	0 .013	—	—
		10	0 .022	0 .022	—	—
		9	0 .037	—	—	—
	5	18	3 .040	2 .006	2 .006	1 .001
		17	2 .021	2 .021	1 .003	1 .003
		16	2 .048	1 .008	1 .008	0 .001
		15	1 .017	1 .017	0 .002	0 .002
		14	1 .033	0 .004	0 .004	0 .004
		13	0 .007	0 .007	0 .007	—
		12	0 .014	0 .014	—	—
		11	0 .024	0 .024	—	—
		10	0 .038	—	—	—
	4	18	2 .026	1 .003	1 .003	1 .003
		17	1 .010−	1 .010−	1 .010−	0 .001
		16	1 .024	1 .024	0 .002	0 .002
		15	1 .046	0 .005−	0 .005−	0 .005−
		14	0 .010−	0 .010−	0 .010−	—

		a_1	Significance Level 0.05 (0.10)	0.025 (0.05)	0.01 (0.02)	0.005 (0.01)
$n_1=18$ $n_2=4$		13	0 .017	0 .017	—	—
		12	0 .029	—	—	—
		11	0 .045+	—	—	—
	3	18	1 .014	1 .014	0 .001	0 .001
		17	1 .041	0 .003	0 .003	0 .003
		16	0 .008	0 .008	0 .008	—
		15	0 .015+	0 .015+	—	—
		14	0 .026	—	—	—
		13	0 .042	—	—	—
	2	18	0 .005+	0 .005+	0 .005+	—
		17	0 .016	0 .016	—	—
		16	0 .032	—	—	—
$n_1=19$ $n_2=19$		19	14 .023	14 .023	13 .010−	12 .004
		18	13 .045−	12 .021	11 .009	10 .004
		17	11 .031	10 .015−	9 .006	8 .003
		16	10 .039	9 .019	8 .009	7 .003
		15	9 .046	8 .022	6 .004	6 .004
		14	8 .050−	7 .024	5 .004	5 .004
		13	6 .025+	5 .011	4 .004	4 .004
		12	5 .024	5 .024	3 .003	3 .003
		11	5 .050−	4 .022	3 .009	2 .003
		10	4 .046	3 .019	2 .006	1 .002
		9	3 .039	2 .015−	1 .004	1 .004
		8	2 .031	1 .009	1 .009	0 .002
		7	1 .021	1 .021	0 .004	0 .004
		6	1 .045−	0 .010−	0 .010−	—
		5	0 .023	0 .023	—	—
	18	19	14 .046	13 .020	12 .008	11 .003
		18	12 .037	11 .017	10 .007	9 .003
		17	10 .024	10 .024	8 .004	8 .004
		16	9 .030	8 .014	7 .006	6 .002
		15	8 .033	7 .015+	6 .006	5 .002
		14	7 .035+	6 .016	5 .006	4 .002
		13	6 .035−	5 .015+	4 .006	3 .002
		12	5 .033	4 .014	3 .005−	3 .005−
		11	4 .030	3 .011	2 .004	2 .004
		10	3 .025−	3 .025−	2 .008	1 .002
		9	3 .049	2 .019	1 .005+	0 .001
		8	2 .038	1 .012	0 .002	0 .002
		7	1 .025+	0 .005−	0 .005−	0 .005−
		6	0 .012	0 .012	—	—
		5	0 .027	—	—	—
	17	19	13 .040	12 .016	11 .006	10 .002
		18	11 .030	10 .013	9 .005+	8 .002
		17	10 .040	9 .018	8 .008	7 .003
		16	9 .047	8 .022	7 .009	6 .003

Appendix Table 5 (Continued)
Tables for Testing Significance in 2 × 2 Tables with Unequal Samples

		a_1	Significance Level 0.05 (0.10)	0.025 (0.05)	0.01 (0.02)	0.005 (0.01)
$n_1 = 19$	$n_2 = 17$	15	8 .050 −	7 .023	6 .010 −	5 .004
		14	6 .023	6 .023	5 .010 −	4 .003
		13	6 .049	5 .022	4 .008	3 .003
		12	5 .045 −	4 .019	3 .007	2 .002
		11	4 .039	3 .015 +	2 .005 −	2 .005 −
		10	3 .032	2 .011	1 .003	1 .003
		9	2 .024	2 .024	1 .007	0 .001
		8	2 .047	1 .015 −	0 .002	0 .002
		7	1 .031	0 .006	0 .006	—
		6	0 .014	0 .014	—	—
		5	0 .031	—	—	—
	16	19	12 .035 −	11 .013	10 .005 −	10 .005 −
		18	10 .024	10 .024	9 .010 −	8 .004
		17	9 .031	8 .013	7 .005 +	6 .002
		16	8 .035 −	7 .015 +	6 .006	5 .002
		15	7 .036	6 .015 +	5 .006	4 .002
		14	6 .034	5 .014	4 .005 +	3 .002
		13	5 .031	4 .012	3 .004	3 .004
		12	4 .027	3 .010 −	3 .010 −	2 .003
		11	3 .021	3 .021	2 .007	1 .002
		10	3 .042	2 .015 −	1 .004	1 .004
		9	2 .030	1 .009	1 .009	0 .001
		8	1 .018	1 .018	0 .003	0 .003
		7	1 .037	0 .007	0 .007	—
		6	0 .017	0 .017	—	—
		5	0 .036	—	—	—
	15	19	11 .029	10 .011	9 .004	9 .004
		18	10 .046	9 .019	8 .007	7 .002
		17	8 .023	8 .023	7 .009	6 .003
		16	7 .025 −	7 .025 −	6 .010 −	5 .003
		15	6 .024	6 .024	5 .009	4 .003
		14	5 .022	5 .022	4 .008	3 .002
		13	5 .045 +	4 .018	3 .006	2 .002
		12	4 .037	3 .014	2 .004	2 .004
		11	3 .029	2 .009	2 .009	1 .002
		10	2 .020	2 .020	1 .005 +	0 .001
		9	2 .039	1 .011	0 .002	0 .002
		8	1 .023	1 .023	0 .004	0 .004
		7	1 .046	0 .009	0 .009	—
		6	0 .020	0 .020	—	—
		5	0 .042	—	—	—
	14	19	10 .024	10 .024	9 .008	8 .003
		18	9 .037	8 .014	7 .005 −	7 .005 −
		17	8 .042	7 .017	6 .006	5 .002
		16	7 .042	6 .017	5 .006	4 .002
		15	6 .039	5 .015 +	4 .005 +	3 .001
		14	5 .034	4 .013	3 .004	3 .004
		13	4 .027	3 .009	3 .009	2 .003
		12	3 .020	3 .020	2 .006	1 .001
		11	3 .040	2 .013	1 .003	1 .003
		10	2 .027	1 .007	1 .007	0 .001
		9	1 .015 −	1 .015 −	0 .002	0 .002
		8	1 .030	0 .005 +	0 .005 +	—
		7	0 .012	0 .012	—	—
		6	0 .024	0 .024	—	—
		5	0 .049	—	—	—
$n_1 = 19$	$n_2 = 13$	19	9 .020	9 .020	8 .006	7 .002
		18	8 .029	7 .010 +	6 .003	6 .003
		17	7 .031	6 .011	5 .004	5 .004
		16	6 .029	5 .011	4 .003	4 .003
		15	5 .025 +	4 .009	4 .009	3 .003
		14	4 .020	4 .020	3 .006	2 .002
		13	4 .041	3 .015 −	2 .004	2 .004
		12	3 .029	2 .009	2 .009	1 .002
		11	2 .019	2 .019	1 .005 −	1 .005 −
		10	2 .036	1 .010 −	1 .010 −	0 .001
		9	1 .020	1 .020	0 .003	0 .003
		8	1 .038	0 .007	0 .007	—
		7	0 .015 −	0 .015 −	—	—
		6	0 .030	—	—	—
	12	19	9 .049	8 .016	7 .005 −	7 .005 −
		18	7 .022	7 .022	6 .007	5 .002
		17	6 .022	6 .022	5 .007	4 .002
		16	5 .019	5 .019	4 .006	3 .002
		15	5 .042	4 .015 +	3 .004	3 .004
		14	4 .032	3 .011	2 .003	2 .003
		13	3 .023	3 .023	2 .006	1 .001
		12	3 .043	2 .014	1 .003	1 .003
		11	2 .027	1 .007	1 .007	0 .001
		10	2 .050 −	1 .014	0 .002	0 .002
		9	1 .027	0 .005 −	0 .005 −	0 .005 −
		8	1 .050 −	0 .010 −	0 .010 −	—
		7	0 .019	0 .019	—	—
		6	0 .037	—	—	—
	11	19	8 .041	7 .012	6 .003	6 .003
		18	7 .047	6 .016	5 .004	5 .004
		17	6 .043	5 .015 −	4 .004	4 .004
		16	5 .035 +	4 .012	3 .003	3 .003
		15	4 .027	3 .008	3 .008	2 .002
		14	3 .018	3 .018	2 .005 −	2 .005 −
		13	3 .035 +	2 .010 +	1 .002	1 .002
		12	2 .021	2 .021	1 .005 −	1 .005 −
		11	2 .040	1 .010 +	0 .001	0 .001
		10	1 .020	1 .020	0 .003	0 .003
		9	1 .037	0 .006	0 .006	—
		8	0 .013	0 .013	—	—
		7	0 .025 −	0 .025 −	—	—
		6	0 .046	—	—	—
	10	19	7 .033	6 .009	6 .009	5 .002
		18	6 .036	5 .011	4 .003	4 .003
		17	5 .030	4 .009	4 .009	3 .002
		16	4 .022	4 .022	3 .006	2 .001
		15	4 .047	3 .015 −	2 .004	2 .004
		14	3 .030	2 .008	2 .008	1 .002
		13	2 .017	2 .017	1 .004	1 .004
		12	2 .033	1 .008	1 .008	0 .001
		11	1 .016	1 .016	0 .002	0 .002
		10	1 .029	0 .005 −	0 .005 −	0 .005 −
		9	0 .009	0 .009	0 .009	—
		8	0 .018	0 .018	—	—
		7	0 .032	—	—	—

Appendix Table 5 (Continued)
Tables for Testing Significance in 2 × 2 Tables with Unequal Samples

Significance Level

	a_1	0.05 (0.10)	0.025 (0.05)	0.01 (0.02)	0.005 (0.01)
$n_1=19$ $n_2=9$ 19	19	6 .026	5 .006	5 .006	4 .001
	18	5 .026	4 .007	4 .007	3 .001
	17	4 .020	4 .020	3 .005 −	3 .005 −
	16	4 .044	3 .013	2 .003	2 .003
	15	3 .028	2 .007	2 .007	1 .001
	14	2 .015 −	2 .015 −	1 .003	1 .003
	13	2 .029	1 .006	1 .006	0 .001
	12	1 .013	1 .013	0 .002	0 .002
	11	1 .024	1 .024	0 .004	0 .004
	10	1 .042	0 .007	0 .007	—
	9	0 .013	0 .013	—	—
	8	0 .024	0 .024	—	—
	7	0 .043	—	—	—
8	19	5 .019	5 .019	4 .004	4 .004
	18	4 .017	4 .017	3 .004	3 .004
	17	4 .044	3 .011	2 .002	2 .002
	16	3 .027	2 .006	2 .006	1 .001
	15	2 .014	2 .014	1 .002	1 .002
	14	2 .027	1 .006	1 .006	0 .001
	13	2 .049	1 .011	0 .001	0 .001
	12	1 .021	1 .021	0 .003	0 .003
	11	1 .038	0 .006	0 .006	—
	10	0 .011	0 .011	—	—
	9	0 .020	0 .020	—	—
	8	0 .034	—	—	—
7	19	4 .013	4 .013	3 .002	3 .002
	18	4 .047	3 .010 +	2 .002	2 .002
	17	3 .028	2 .006	2 .006	1 .001
	16	2 .014	2 .014	1 .002	1 .002
	15	2 .028	1 .005 +	1 .005 +	0 .001
	14	1 .011	1 .011	0 .001	0 .001
	13	1 .021	1 .021	0 .003	0 .003
	12	1 .037	0 .005 +	0 .005 +	—
	11	0 .010 −	0 .010 −	0 .010 −	—
	10	0 .017	0 .017	—	—
	9	0 .030	—	—	—
	8	0 .048	—	—	—
6	19	4 .050	3 .009	3 .009	2 .001
	18	3 .031	2 .005 +	2 .005 +	1 .001
	17	2 .015 +	2 .015 +	1 .002	1 .002
	16	2 .032	1 .006	1 .006	0 .000
	15	1 .012	1 .012	0 .001	0 .001
	14	1 .023	1 .023	0 .003	0 .003
	13	1 .039	0 .005 +	0 .005 +	—
	12	0 .010 −	0 .010 −	0 .010 −	—
	11	0 .017	0 .017	—	—
	10	0 .028	—	—	—
	9	0 .045 +	—	—	—
5	19	3 .036	2 .005 −	2 .005 −	2 .005 −
	18	2 .018	2 .018	1 .002	1 .002
	17	2 .042	1 .006	1 .006	0 .000
	16	1 .014	1 .014	0 .001	0 .001
	15	1 .028	0 .003	0 .003	0 .003
	14	1 .047	0 .006	0 .006	—
	13	0 .011	0 .011	—	—

Significance Level

	a_1	0.05 (0.10)	0.025 (0.05)	0.01 (0.02)	0.005 (0.01)
$n_1=19$ $n_2=5$ 12	12	0 .019	0 .019	—	—
	11	0 .030	—	—	—
	10	0 .047	—	—	—
4	19	2 .024	2 .024	1 .002	1 .002
	18	1 .009	1 .009	1 .009	0 .001
	17	1 .021	1 .021	0 .002	0 .002
	16	1 .040	0 .004	0 .004	0 .004
	15	0 .008	0 .008	0 .008	—
	14	0 .014	0 .014	—	—
	13	0 .024	0 .024	—	—
	12	0 .037	—	—	—
3	19	1 .013	1 .013	0 .001	0 .001
	18	1 .038	0 .003	0 .003	0 .003
	17	0 .006	0 .006	0 .006	—
	16	0 .013	0 .013	—	—
	15	0 .023	0 .023	—	—
	14	0 .036	—	—	—
2	19	0 .005 −	0 .005 −	0 .005 −	0 .005
	18	0 .014	0 .014	—	—
	17	0 .029	—	—	—
	16	0 .048	—	—	—
$n_1=20$ $n_2=20$ 20	20	15 .024	15 .024	13 .004	13 .004
	19	14 .046	13 .022	12 .010 −	11 .004
	18	12 .032	11 .015 +	10 .007	9 .003
	17	11 .041	10 .020	9 .009	8 .004
	16	10 .048	9 .024	7 .005 −	7 .005
	15	8 .027	7 .012	6 .005 +	5 .002
	14	7 .028	6 .013	5 .005 +	4 .002
	13	6 .028	5 .012	4 .005 −	4 .005
	12	5 .027	4 .011	3 .004	3 .004
	11	4 .024	3 .009	2 .003	2 .003
	10	4 .048	3 .020	2 .007	1 .002
	9	3 .041	2 .015 +	1 .004	1 .004
	8	2 .032	1 .010 −	1 .010 −	0 .002
	7	1 .022	1 .022	0 .004	0 .004
	6	1 .046	0 .010 +	—	—
	5	0 .024	0 .024	—	—
19	20	15 .047	14 .020	13 .008	12 .003
	19	13 .039	12 .018	11 .008	10 .003
	18	11 .026	10 .012	9 .005 −	9 .005 −
	17	10 .032	9 .015 −	8 .006	7 .002
	16	9 .036	8 .017	7 .007	6 .003
	15	8 .038	7 .018	6 .008	5 .003
	14	7 .039	6 .018	5 .007	4 .003
	13	6 .038	5 .017	4 .007	3 .002
	12	5 .035 +	4 .015 +	3 .005 +	2 .002
	11	4 .031	3 .012	2 .004	2 .004
	10	3 .026	2 .009	2 .009	1 .002
	9	2 .019	2 .019	1 .005 +	0 .002
	8	2 .039	1 .012	0 .002	0 .002
	7	1 .026	0 .005 +	0 .005 +	—
	6	0 .012	0 .012	—	—
	5	0 .027	—	—	—

Tables for Testing Significance in 2 × 2 Tables with Unequal Samples

Left panel — $n_1 = 20$, $n_2 = 18$

	a_1	Significance Level 0.05 (0.10)	0.025 (0.05)	0.01 (0.02)	0.005 (0.01)
20	20	14 .041	13 .017	12 .007	11 .003
	19	12 .032	11 .014	10 .006	9 .002
	18	11 .043	10 .020	9 .008	8 .003
	17	10 .050 −	9 .024	7 .004	7 .004
	16	8 .026	7 .011	6 .005 −	6 .005 −
	15	7 .027	6 .012	5 .004	5 .004
	14	6 .026	5 .011	4 .004	4 .004
	13	5 .024	5 .024	4 .009	3 .003
	12	5 .047	4 .020	3 .007	2 .002
	11	4 .041	3 .016	2 .005 +	1 .001
	10	3 .033	2 .012	1 .003	1 .003
	9	2 .024	2 .024	1 .007	0 .001
	8	2 .048	1 .015 −	0 .003	0 .003
	7	1 .031	0 .006	0 .006	—
	6	0 .014	0 .014	—	—
	5	0 .031	—	—	—
17	20	13 .036	12 .014	11 .005 +	10 .002
	19	11 .026	10 .011	9 .004	9 .004
	18	10 .034	9 .015 −	8 .006	7 .002
	17	9 .038	8 .017	7 .007	6 .003
	16	8 .040	7 .018	6 .007	5 .003
	15	7 .039	6 .017	5 .007	4 .002
	14	6 .037	5 .016	4 .006	3 .002
	13	5 .033	4 .013	3 .005 −	3 .005 −
	12	4 .028	3 .010 +	2 .003	2 .003
	11	3 .022	3 .022	2 .007	1 .002
	10	3 .042	2 .015 +	1 .004	1 .004
	9	2 .031	1 .009	1 .009	0 .001
	8	1 .019	1 .019	0 .003	0 .003
	7	1 .037	0 .008	0 .008	—
	6	0 .017	0 .017	—	—
	5	0 .036	—	—	—
16	20	12 .031	11 .012	10 .004	10 .004
	19	11 .049	10 .021	9 .008	8 .003
	18	9 .026	8 .011	7 .004	7 .004
	17	8 .028	7 .012	6 .004	6 .004
	16	7 .028	6 .012	5 .004	5 .004
	15	6 .026	5 .011	4 .004	4 .004
	14	5 .023	5 .023	4 .009	3 .003
	13	5 .046	4 .019	3 .007	2 .002
	12	4 .038	3 .014	2 .004	2 .004
	11	3 .029	2 .010 −	2 .010 −	1 .002
	10	2 .020	2 .020	1 .005 +	0 .001
	9	2 .039	1 .011	0 .002	0 .002
	8	1 .023	1 .023	0 .004	0 .004
	7	1 .045 +	0 .009	0 .009	—
	6	0 .020	0 .020	—	—
	5	0 .041	—	—	—
15	20	11 .026	10 .009	10 .009	9 .003
	19	10 .040	9 .016	8 .006	7 .002
	18	9 .046	8 .019	7 .007	6 .002
	17	8 .047	7 .020	6 .008	5 .003
	16	7 .045 −	6 .019	5 .007	4 .002
	15	6 .040	5 .017	4 .006	3 .002
	14	5 .034	4 .013	3 .004	3 .004

Right panel — $n_1 = 20$, $n_2 = 15$

	a_1	Significance Level 0.05 (0.10)	0.025 (0.05)	0.01 (0.02)	0.005 (0.01)
13	13	4 .028	3 .010 −	3 .010 −	2 .003
	12	3 .020	3 .020	2 .006	1 .001
	11	3 .039	2 .013	1 .003	1 .003
	10	2 .026	1 .007	1 .007	0 .001
	9	2 .049	1 .015 −	0 .002	0 .002
	8	1 .029	0 .005 +	0 .005 +	—
	7	0 .012	0 .012	—	—
	6	0 .024	0 .024	—	—
	5	0 .048	—	—	—
14	20	10 .022	10 .022	9 .007	8 .002
	19	9 .032	8 .012	7 .004	7 .004
	18	8 .035 +	7 .014	6 .005 −	6 .005 −
	17	7 .035 −	6 .013	5 .005 −	5 .005 −
	16	6 .031	5 .012	4 .004	4 .004
	15	5 .026	4 .009	4 .009	3 .003
	14	4 .020	4 .020	3 .007	2 .002
	13	4 .040	3 .015 −	2 .004	2 .004
	12	3 .029	2 .009	2 .009	1 .002
	11	2 .018	2 .018	1 .005 −	1 .005 −
	10	2 .035 +	1 .010 −	1 .010 −	0 .001
	9	1 .019	1 .019	0 .003	0 .003
	8	1 .037	0 .007	0 .007	—
	7	0 .014	0 .014	—	—
	6	0 .029	—	—	—
13	20	9 .017	9 .017	8 .005 +	7 .002
	19	8 .025 −	8 .025 −	7 .008	6 .003
	18	7 .026	6 .009	6 .009	5 .003
	17	6 .024	6 .024	5 .008	4 .002
	16	5 .020	5 .020	4 .007	3 .002
	15	5 .041	4 .015 +	3 .005 −	3 .005 −
	14	4 .031	3 .011	2 .003	2 .003
	13	3 .022	3 .022	2 .006	1 .001
	12	3 .041	2 .013	1 .003	1 .003
	11	2 .026	1 .007	1 .007	0 .001
	10	2 .047	1 .013	0 .002	0 .002
	9	1 .026	0 .004	0 .004	0 .004
	8	1 .047	0 .009	0 .009	—
	7	0 .018	0 .018	—	—
	6	0 .035 −	—	—	—
12	20	9 .044	8 .014	7 .004	7 .004
	19	7 .018	7 .018	6 .006	5 .002
	18	6 .018	6 .018	5 .006	4 .002
	17	6 .043	5 .016	4 .005 −	4 .005 −
	16	5 .034	4 .012	3 .003	3 .003
	15	4 .025 +	3 .008	3 .008	2 .002
	14	4 .049	3 .017	2 .005 −	2 .005 −
	13	3 .033	2 .010 −	2 .010 −	1 .002
	12	2 .020	2 .020	1 .005 −	1 .005 −
	11	2 .036	1 .009	1 .009	0 .001
	10	1 .018	1 .018	0 .003	0 .003
	9	1 .034	0 .006	0 .006	—
	8	0 .012	0 .012	—	—
	7	0 .023	0 .023	—	—
	6	0 .043	—	—	—

Appendix Table 5 (Continued)
Tables for Testing Significance in 2 × 2 Tables with Unequal Samples

$n_1 = 20$

n_2	a_1	Significance Level 0.05 (0.10)	0.025 (0.05)	0.01 (0.02)	0.005 (0.01)
11	20	8 .037	7 .010 +	6 .003	6 .003
	19	7 .042	6 .013	5 .004	5 .004
	18	6 .037	5 .012	4 .003	4 .003
	17	5 .029	4 .009	4 .009	3 .002
	16	4 .021	4 .021	3 .006	2 .001
	15	4 .042	3 .014	2 .003	2 .003
	14	3 .028	2 .008	2 .008	1 .001
	13	2 .016	2 .016	1 .003	1 .003
	12	2 .029	1 .007	1 .007	0 .001
	11	1 .014	1 .014	0 .002	0 .002
	10	1 .026	0 .004	0 .004	0 .004
	9	1 .046	0 .008	0 .008	—
	8	0 .016	0 .016	—	—
	7	0 .029	—	—	—
10	20	7 .030	6 .008	6 .008	5 .002
	19	6 .031	5 .009	5 .009	4 .002
	18	5 .026	4 .007	4 .007	3 .002
	17	4 .018	4 .018	3 .005 −	3 .005 −
	16	4 .039	3 .012	2 .003	2 .003
	15	3 .024	3 .024	2 .006	1 .001
	14	3 .045 +	2 .013	1 .003	1 .003
	13	2 .025 +	1 .006	1 .006	0 .001
	12	2 .045 −	1 .011	0 .001	0 .001
	11	1 .021	1 .021	0 .003	0 .003
	10	1 .037	0 .006	0 .006	—
	9	0 .012	0 .012	—	—
	8	0 .022	0 .022	—	—
	7	0 .038	—	—	—
9	20	6 .023	6 .023	5 .005 +	4 .001
	19	5 .022	5 .022	4 .005 +	3 .001
	18	4 .016	4 .016	3 .004	3 .004
	17	4 .037	3 .010 +	2 .002	2 .002
	16	3 .022	3 .022	2 .005 +	1 .001
	15	3 .043	2 .012	1 .002	1 .002
	14	2 .023	2 .023	1 .005 −	1 .005 −
	13	2 .041	1 .009	1 .009	0 .001
	12	1 .018	1 .018	0 .002	0 .002
	11	1 .032	0 .005 −	0 .005 −	0 .005 −
	10	0 .009	0 .009	0 .009	—
	9	0 .017	0 .017	—	—
	8	0 .029	—	—	—
	7	0 .050 −	—	—	—
8	20	5 .017	5 .017	4 .003	4 .003
	19	4 .015 −	4 .015 −	3 .003	3 .003
	18	4 .038	3 .009	3 .009	2 .002
	17	3 .022	3 .022	2 .005 −	2 .005 −
	16	3 .044	2 .011	1 .002	1 .002
	15	2 .022	2 .022	1 .004	1 .004
	14	2 .040	1 .009	1 .009	0 .001
	13	1 .016	1 .016	0 .002	0 .002
	12	1 .029	0 .004	0 .004	0 .004
	11	1 .048	0 .008	0 .008	—
	10	0 .014	0 .014	—	—
	9	0 .024	0 .024	—	—
	8	0 .041	—	—	—

$n_1 = 20$

n_2	a_1	Significance Level 0.05 (0.10)	0.025 (0.05)	0.01 (0.02)	0.005 (0.01)
7	20	4 .012	4 .012	3 .002	3 .002
	19	4 .042	3 .009	3 .009	2 .001
	18	3 .024	3 .024	2 .005 −	2 .005 −
	17	3 .050 −	2 .011	1 .002	1 .002
	16	2 .023	2 .023	1 .004	1 .004
	15	2 .043	1 .009	1 .009	0 .001
	14	1 .016	1 .016	0 .002	0 .002
	13	1 .029	0 .004	0 .004	0 .004
	12	1 .048	0 .007	0 .007	—
	11	0 .013	0 .013	—	—
	10	0 .022	0 .022	—	—
	9	0 .036	—	—	—
6	20	4 .046	3 .008	3 .008	2 .001
	19	3 .028	2 .005 −	2 .005 −	2 .005 −
	18	2 .013	2 .013	1 .002	1 .002
	17	2 .028	1 .004	1 .004	1 .004
	16	1 .010 −	1 .010 −	1 .010 −	0 .001
	15	1 .018	1 .018	0 .002	0 .002
	14	1 .032	0 .004	0 .004	0 .004
	13	0 .007	0 .007	0 .007	—
	12	0 .013	0 .013	—	—
	11	0 .022	0 .022	—	—
	10	0 .035 −	—	—	—
5	20	3 .033	2 .004	2 .004	2 .004
	19	2 .016	2 .016	1 .002	1 .002
	18	2 .038	1 .005 +	1 .005 +	0 .000
	17	1 .012	1 .012	0 .001	0 .001
	16	1 .023	1 .023	0 .002	0 .002
	15	1 .040	0 .005 −	0 .005 −	0 .005 −
	14	0 .009	0 .009	0 .009	—
	13	0 .015 −	0 .015 −	—	—
	12	0 .024	0 .024	—	—
	11	0 .038	—	—	—
4	20	2 .022	2 .022	1 .002	1 .002
	19	1 .008	1 .008	1 .008	0 .000
	18	1 .018	1 .018	0 .001	0 .001
	17	1 .035 +	0 .003	0 .003	0 .003
	16	0 .007	0 .007	0 .007	—
	15	0 .012	0 .012	—	—
	14	0 .020	0 .020	—	—
	13	0 .031	—	—	—
	12	0 .047	—	—	—
3	20	1 .012	1 .012	0 .001	0 .001
	19	1 .034	0 .002	0 .002	0 .002
	18	0 .006	0 .006	0 .006	—
	17	0 .011	0 .011	—	—
	16	0 .020	0 .020	—	—
	15	0 .032	—	—	—
	14	0 .047	—	—	—
2	20	0 .004	0 .004	0 .004	0 .004
	19	0 .013	0 .013	—	—
	18	0 .026	—	—	—
	17	0 .043	—	—	—
1	20	0 .048	—	—	—

Appendix Table 6
Cumulative Normal Distribution

Location of Vertical Line	Area	Location of Vertical Line	Area
$\mu - 3.00\ \sigma$	.001	$\mu +\ .00\ \sigma$	.500
$\mu - 2.75\ \sigma$	.003	$\mu +\ .25\ \sigma$	.599
$\mu - 2.50\ \sigma$	.006	$\mu +\ .50\ \sigma$	.692
$\mu - 2.25\ \sigma$	.012	$\mu +\ .75\ \sigma$	.773
$\mu - 2.00\ \sigma$	.023	$\mu + 1.00\ \sigma$	.841
$\mu - 1.75\ \sigma$	.040	$\mu + 1.25\ \sigma$	.894
$\mu - 1.50\ \sigma$	.067	$\mu + 1.50\ \sigma$	.933
$\mu - 1.25\ \sigma$	.106	$\mu + 1.75\ \sigma$	.960
$\mu - 1.00\ \sigma$	.159	$\mu + 2.00\ \sigma$	.977
$\mu -\ .75\ \sigma$	.227	$\mu + 2.25\ \sigma$	.988
$\mu -\ .50\ \sigma$	.308	$\mu + 2.50\ \sigma$	.994
$\mu -\ .25\ \sigma$	.401	$\mu + 2.75\ \sigma$	.997
$\mu -\ .00\ \sigma$	.500	$\mu + 3.00\ \sigma$	.999

Note: The area column figure is the percentage of the total area under a normal distribution curve to the left of a vertical line indicated by the mean ± standard deviation column (see Figs. 4-1 and 4-2). Text Explanation: pages 18, 19, 20, 21, 22, 23.

Appendix Table 7
Factors for Computing One-Sided Confidence Limits for σ

Degrees of Freedom ν	$A_{.05}$	$A_{.95}$	$A_{.025}$	$A_{.975}$	$A_{.01}$	$A_{.99}$	$A_{.005}$	$A_{.995}$
1	.5103	15.947	.4461	31.910	.3882	79.786	.3562	159.576
2	.5778	4.415	.5207	6.285	.4660	9.975	.4344	14.124
3	.6196	2.920	.5665	3.729	.5142	5.111	.4834	6.467
4	.6493	2.372	.5992	2.874	.5489	3.669	.5188	4.396
5	.6721	2.089	.6242	2.453	.5757	3.003	.5464	3.485
6	.6903	1.915	.6444	2.202	.5974	2.623	.5688	2.980
7	.7054	1.797	.6612	2.035	.6155	2.377	.5875	2.660
8	.7183	1.711	.6754	1.916	.6310	2.204	.6037	2.439
9	.7293	1.645	.6878	1.826	.6445	2.076	.6177	2.278
10	.7391	1.593	.6987	1.755	.6564	1.977	.6301	2.154
11	.7477	1.551	.7084	1.698	.6670	1.898	.6412	2.056
12	.7554	1.515	.7171	1.651	.6765	1.833	.6512	1.976
13	.7624	1.485	.7250	1.611	.6852	1.779	.6603	1.909
14	.7688	1.460	.7321	1.577	.6931	1.733	.6686	1.854
15	.7747	1.437	.7387	1.548	.7004	1.694	.6762	1.806
20	.7979	1.358	.7650	1.444	.7297	1.556	.7071	1.640
25	.8149	1.308	.7843	1.380	.7511	1.473	.7299	1.542
30	.8279	1.274	.7991	1.337	.7678	1.416	.7477	1.475
40	.8470	1.228	.8210	1.279	.7925	1.343	.7740	1.390
50	.8606	1.199	.8367	1.243	.8103	1.297	.7931	1.337
60	.8710	1.179	.8487	1.217	.8239	1.265	.8078	1.299
70	.8793	1.163	.8583	1.198	.8349	1.241	.8196	1.272
80	.8861	1.151	.8662	1.183	.8439	1.222	.8293	1.250
90	.8919	1.141	.8728	1.171	.8515	1.207	.8376	1.233
100	.8968	1.133	.8785	1.161	.8581	1.195	.8446	1.219

Source: M. G. Natrella, *Experimental Statistics*. National Bureau of Standards Handbook 91, Table 21A (Washington, D.C.: U.S. Government Printing Office, 1976).
Text Explanation: pages 18, 181.

Annotated General Bibliography

Annotated General Bibliography

Colton, T. *Statistics in Medicine*. Boston: Little, Brown, 1974. A good introduction to common types of statistical thinking and practice relevant to medical subjects.

Dixon, W. J., and Massey, F. J., Jr. *Introduction to Statistical Analysis* (3rd ed.). New York: McGraw-Hill, 1969. $10.95. This is an excellent basic textbook in statistics, planned for a one-year college course meeting three times a week. The new edition represents a considerable improvement over the earlier ones in having a better format, more tables, and clearer expositions. Very mathematical.

Fisher, R. A., and Yates, F. *Statistical Tables for Biological, Agricultural and Medical Research* (6th ed., rev. and enlarged). New York: Hafner, 1974. $7.95. Contains many comprehensive tables used in various types of research.

Gabrieli, E. R. (Ed.). *The Use of Data Mechanization and Computers in Clinical Medicine*. Annals of the New York Academy of Sciences, Vol. 161, Art. 2, Sept. 30, 1969. (N.Y. Academy of Sciences, 2 East 63rd Street, New York 10021.) Contains a wide variety of articles dealing with the interface of medical practice, laboratories, statistics, and computers.

Moroney, M. J. *Facts from Figures*. Pelican Book A236 (paperback). Baltimore: Penguin Books, 1956. $2.50. A general exposition of useful statistics. An unusually good buy.

Natrella, M. G. *Experimental Statistics* (National Bureau of Standards Handbook 91), 1963, reprinted 1976. Available from Superintendent of Documents, U.S. Government Printing Office, Washington, D. C. 20402. An excellent volume with comprehensive tables and lucid examples.

Wilcoxon, F., Katti, S. K., and Wilcox, R. A. *Critical Values and Probability Levels for the Wilcoxon Rank Sum Test and the Wilcoxon Signed Rank Test*, 1963. Prepared and distributed by Lederle Laboratories Division, American Cyanamid Co., Pearl River, N.Y. 10965. Available without charge at this time. Invaluable tables for rank-sum and signed-rank test.

Youden, W. J. *Statistical Methods for Chemists*. New York and London: John Wiley & Sons, 1951. $9.25. A standard work, small and lucidly written.

Youden, W. J., and Steiner, E. H. *Statistical Techniques for Collaborative Tests*. Association of Official Analytical Chemists, 1975. Available from Association of Official Analytical Chemists, Box 540, Benjamin Franklin Station, Washington, D. C. 20044.

Index

Index